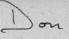

Secrets To A
Healthy Heart
And Low Cholesterol

Secrets To A Healthy Heart And Low Cholesterol

Proven guidelines and documented facts for the natural self-treatment and prevention of heart disease, high cholesterol, and other related ailments in conjunction with the world-famous breakthrough formula by Prof. Flemming Norgaard, M.D., D.D.S.

Fischer Publishing Corporation
Canfield, Ohio 44406

Secrets To A Healthy Heart
And Low Cholesterol

Proven guidelines and documented facts for the natural self-treatment and prevention of heart disease, high cholesterol, and other related ailments in conjunction with the world-famous breakthrough formula by Prof. Flemming Norgaard, M.D., D.D.S.

ISBN 0-915421-13-5

Printed in the United States of America

FISCHER PUBLISHING CORPORATION
Canfield, Ohio 44406

Disclaimer

This book is informational only and should not be considered as a substitute for consultation with a duly-licensed medical doctor. Any attempt to diagnose and treat an illness should come under the direction of a physician. The author is not himself a medical doctor and does not purport to offer medical advice, make diagnoses, prescribe remedies for specific medical conditions or substitute for medical consultation.

Nothing noted in the text should be considered an attempt by William L. Fischer or the publisher to practice medicine, prescribe remedies, make diagnoses, or act as persuasion for enforcing some mode of surgery. Instead, knowledge received is strictly for purposes of education, and William L. Fischer takes no responsibility for its content.

Table of Contents

INTRODUCTION

Few of us are not concerned about the health of our heart or our cholesterol level. Just about every day, I meet a friend who has been told by his doctor that his cholesterol level is too high. It usually comes as a shock to them.

Perhaps you are among these people who are now keenly aware of their problem, because your doctor has told you to lower it. Or perhaps you've been listening to news reports and realize the importance of keeping it within healthy bounds, but are a little confused about how to do it.

Secrets to a Healthy Heart and Low Cholesterol was written for you. This book can be your valued partner in lowering or maintaining your cholesterol level. You will learn about cholesterol, what it does, how it works and why too much is dangerous. It will also show you how to take positive steps in improving your current situation and maintaining it for life long health.

Hardening of the arteries, or atherosclerosis, is also discussed in detail. Too many of us are walking around with advanced cases of this disease, and we don't even know it. It gives no warning signals until it is almost too late. There are effective measures you can take to help delay or even prevent the onset of this very serious health problem.

Your heart is the most remarkable muscle of your body. It's incredibly durable. It works constantly — 24 hours a day, 7 days a week — without rest. Without your heart pumping blood throughout your body, life would be impossible.

Yet, we seldom give it much thought — unless something goes wrong with it.

Think of your heart in the same way you would think of your car—as a piece of fine machinery which needs basic preventive maintenance. We all know the importance of oil changes for our automobile, new spark plugs and other items which ensure the car runs smoothly.

Do the same for your heart. Provide it with sound healthy habits and it will give you a lifetime of fine performance.

It's all in your hands. If you follow the guidelines provided in this book, you will have won half of the battle. You owe it to yourself and your loved ones to take the best possible care. We must emphasize prevention is the best alternative.

This book demonstrates the most efficient ways to regain or maintain your health.

Use it wisely.

To your good health
William L. Fischer

Chapter 1

The Heart and How It Works

The American Heart Association estimates that about 1.5 million people in this country will suffer heart attacks this year. Of those, approximately 540,000 will die as a result, most of whom never reach the hospital for medical treatment.

Moreover, it is estimated that more than 30 million people have some form of heart disease which costs the nation about 40 million dollars annually in terms of treatment and loss of productivity.

While these statistics are grim, they are improving. Today, through the combination of advanced medical technology and increasing knowledge concerning preventive measures, the incidence of deaths due to heart disease is decreasing. About 100,000 less people die yearly now than did a decade ago.

This, of course, is good news, but it should not lull the public into a false sense of security.

Heart disease is a major killer.

1

The heart attack is a relatively new health problem in medical history, the first one not being recorded until the early 20th century. The year was 1912 and the attack was suffered by a 55-year-old banker from Chicago, Ill. The diagnosis met with ridicule from many medical professionals, even though an autopsy report confirmed the cause of death.

Some 75 years later the diagnosis of heart attack is too common as are its major symptoms—hardening of the arteries and high blood pressure.

To understand the development of heart disease one first must understand how the heart and the cardiovascular system works.

How the Heart Works

The cornerstone of the cardiovascular system is the heart. It's continual pumping provides the blood which flows through the arteries and carries nutrients to every part of the body.

It's a small organ, only about the size of your fist. A normal adult heart weighs about 11 ounces. In a highly-trained athlete, however, it may weigh as much as one pound. The heart is locate between the lungs with its top tilted toward the right side of the body.

Most of the human heart is composed of muscle, called *myocardium*, which is securely placed between a protective inner and outer layer, called endocardium and epicadium, respectively.

Cardiac muscle tissue is unlike any other in the body. It is the only muscle which spontaneously contracts on its own, without any stimulation from the central nervous or hormonal systems.

The heart is actually a "double pump" with four chambers. As it beats, the myocardium pumps blood from the heart through the blood vessels. Between beats, the heart rests only a fraction of a second.

The two pumps of the heart work in harmony. The left side pumps blood throughout the circulatory system. After all areas of the body have been fed with the nutrients and oxygen, the blood returns and is received by the right part of the heart. It sends the blood to the lungs for cleansing. It is here that the waste gas—carbon dioxide—is eliminated and fresh oxygen is received. The left heart uses this "re-nourished" blood with a new load of oxygen and nutrients to circulate through the body again.

A small node in the upper chamber of the heart activates the re-nourished process. It's best described as an electronic impulse center and regu-

3

lates the heart to an average of 60 to 80 beats per minute. Moreover, this node emits electrical pulses which are passed through the body's nervous system, determining the rhythm of the entire circulatory system. In effect, this "pacemaker" sets your pulse.

Heart disease, therefore, can apply to different types of ailments or conditions which would not only affect the heart, but the circulatory system as well, which is dependent upon the heart's consistent pumping to supply blood and nutrients to all the organs of the body.

THE HUMAN HEART

The heart, a four-chambered double pump, beats 100,000 times a day moving 4,300 gallons of oxygen-rich blood through the body's circulatory system.

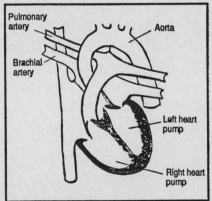

As the heart beats, contractions of the thick muscle wall (myocardium) pump blood from the heart through 60,000 miles of blood vessels. It rests only a fraction of a second between

4

beats.

The right heart pump receives the body's blood after it has delivered nutrients and oxygen to the body tissues. It then sends the blood along the lungs for cleansing. Waste gas is gotten rid of and fresh oxygen is substituted.

The left heart receives this re-nourished blood from the lungs and pumps it through the circulatory system to its eventual return to the right heart.

Heart Failure

The term heart failure sounds as if it refers to a heart which has stopped, but it doesn't. It is the description medical professionals use in reference to a heart which is not functioning effectively.

There are two kinds of heart failure-left sided and right sided. When the left side of the heart is affected, blood accumulates in the veins instead of being carried from the lungs, causing the lungs to fill with fluid.

The symptoms of this type of heart failure are difficulty breathing and a "bubbling" sound as you exhale or inhale. Fatigue may also be a symptom.

Accumulation of blood occurs in the veins leading from other parts of your body to your heart in

5

the case of right sided heart failure. This causes the lower parts of your body to swell. Most often the swelling will affect the legs and ankles. Some people affected with right sided heart failure complain of a persistent cold, dry cough, along with wheezing. Many times this symptom is mistaken for those of an allergic reaction.

Heart failure, in most cases, can be controlled with a *low-salt diet and rest,* as well as medication to remove the fluid from your tissues, dilate your blood vessels and control the heart's contraction.

The Symptoms of A Heart Attack

The common view of a heart attack, usually held by those who have never suffered from one, is that of sudden, severe pain. That is partially right. The attack itself is extremely severe. But many heart attack victims experience a series of less severe symptoms prior to an attack. In fact, some people mistakenly assume they have indigestion, when they are really experiencing the first signals of an impending heart attack.

Angina is one of these symptoms. When one feels an angina pain, it is an advance signal of a heart attack. It is a severe chest pain originating in the heart and usually develops while a person is exercising or under emotional stress. It may also be caused by exposure to the cold or, in fact, any situation which increases the heart's work load, thus, causing an increase in the oxygen supply.

Angina pectoris, its full name, occurs because oxygen requirements exceed the supply available. The heart, in effect, needs more blood than it is receiving. The organ reacts by releasing chemicals which cause pain. Angina develops in a person whose coronary arteries are partly blocked by fatty deposits and are working at only about 40 percent of the normal capacity.

Once the excessive oxygen demand is decreased, blood flow and oxygen availability are restored within five to fifteen minutes—and the pain disappears.

Why Does Angina Occur?

Currently, there are two known reasons why a person develops *angina pectoris.* The first is that a partially blocked vessel cannot meet the oxygen needs of the heart during physical exercise. While the oxygen supply is adequate when the person is at rest, it is not enough when the body engages in physical activity. The heart pumps harder to supply the oxygen, but because of the partial blockage, it is still not enough.

Therefore, the heart muscle releases pain-in-

7

ducing chemicals, in an attempt to halt the activity. When the person rests, the oxygen requirement naturally falls and the heart stops production of the chemicals, which eases the pain. Not too long ago, medical experts believed this to be the only cause of angina. Now they recognize a second cause, but believe it may be an even more important than this one.

Angina can be caused by a muscle spasm in the coronary arteries in response to either *lack of oxygen* or to *stress*. In many cases, even without engaging in physical activity, a person may have angina pain. It is instead prompted by an emotionally upsetting or extremely tense situation.

In these instances the nerves of the heart release the chemicals which cause a spasm in the artery. The spasm, in turn, reduces the flow of blood, which will eventually prompt an angina pain.

The Destruction The Heart Attack Causes

The path of destruction of the industrialized world's greatest killer—the heart attack—is outlined below.

First, the fats in the blood collect inside the coronary arteries, slowly and eventually choking the vessels, which also starve the heart muscle or the *myocardium.*

The areas of starvation are indicated by the darker areas of the diagram, below. The left drawing (No. 1.) shows a partial blockage by a fatty lump on an artery wall.

The blood clot, which normally is a lifesaving property of blood, makes the condition even worse in this instance. Clots form around some of the plaque, and if the combination becomes large enough, the artery is completely plugged and the blood flow is stopped. This is shown in the drawing at the right (No. 2) . The insert shows the plaque and the clot. A much larger portion of muscle, as illustrated by the darkened areas, is starved.

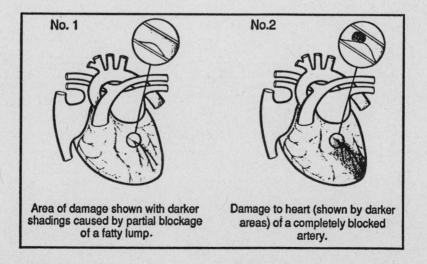

No. 1

No.2

Area of damage shown with darker shadings caused by partial blockage of a fatty lump.

Damage to heart (shown by darker areas) of a completely blocked artery.

9

The third illustration (no. 3) shows the portion of the heart muscle which has been killed by the attack. Scar tissue slowly replaces the dead muscle, a process which takes three to six weeks. The portion of the heart which has been untouched by the experience (which is the lighter areas on the diagram), therefore, must work harder to compensate for the dead areas.

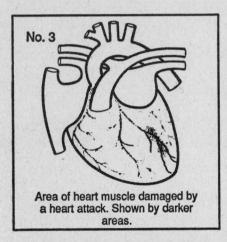

No. 3

Area of heart muscle damaged by a heart attack. Shown by darker areas.

Medical experts believe that a spasm may also play a crucial role in causing angina pain during physical exercise as well. When a person exercises, a spasm may occur in response to the increased oxygen supply. The best evidence, medical experts say, is the use of nitrites to ease angina pain. Nitrites are powerful spasm relievers and most people can inhale, suck or swallow nitrites and rid themselves of the angina.

Many times, especially in the early stages of an angina attack, the pain is often misunderstood. Because the heart is located slightly to the left of the chest, many people expect to feel pain under their left breast. This is not the case, however. One feels angina pain in the *center of the chest,* underneath the breast bone.

The pain usually then spreads to the left shoulder, into the teeth and jaw area, and sometimes even into the wrist. Moreover, angina may occur in the arm, wrist and jaw region without the person ever experiencing pain in the chest. *Angina pain almost always occurs during periods of exercise or stress.*

The Heart Attack

If the blockage of blood flow to the heart is prolonged, then it causes an abnormal heart rhythm, called a *cardiac arrhythmia,* which may advance to a more serious condition called *ventricular fibrillation.* This results in a rapid, extremely ineffective heart beat, where blood is not pumped out of the heart to supply the body. The brain cannot survive for more than four to six minutes without blood and oxygen.

The most successful way of restoring natural rhythm is through electric shock to the heart with use of a machine called a *defibrillator.* If the fibrillation does not begin at once, the person becomes conscious of very intense pain. It is usually much more severe than angina pain and will not disappear with rest. In some cases the pain may last for several hours. The person sweats, turns pale, and has a sense of impending doom. Frequently, dizziness, fainting, nausea and vomiting are also experienced. The pain is an indication that the vessel is completely blocked. If the artery is not opened, the heart muscle will die within a few hours and will be replaced by fibrous tissue. The death of the muscle is called *infarction.*

The recovery chances depend upon the amount of heart muscle lost. If only a small part of the muscle has died, he may be able to function almost normally. If however, a large amount of muscle was lost, any type of exercise may be impossible, because the heart will not be able to provide enough oxygen. If enough muscle was killed during the heart attack that the heart cannot provide for the needs of the body even when resting, death will occur shortly following the attack.

The risk of fibrillation is high during the first hour following an attack. This makes it extremely urgent that a person seek medical aid as soon as possible. The main function of a hospital's coronary care unit is, in fact, to reverse fibrillation immediately with the use of a defibrillator and specific drugs.

The Causes of a Heart Attack

While medical professionals know that an interruption of the blood flow to the heart causes a heart attack, they still don't know what prompts this blockage. Scientists, however, are learning more every day about the causes. In fact, within the last several years, many commonly accepted theories have been replaced with newer ideas, based on research which is producing a fuller understanding of the heart and its arteries.

Medical experts now espouse for possible causes for the occurrence of heart attacks.

1) *The lodging of a piece of solid material (an embolus) in a coronary artery.*

   Lumps may occur when platelets, small cells needed for blood clot formation, stick together and form a thrombus. A thrombus may form in the heart if the valves are not functioning properly. It is then pushed out of the heart into the circulating bloodstream where it can lodge itself in a coronary artery, causing a heart attack. This was once thought to be the primary cause of attacks. Scientists now know, however, that this occurs infrequently.

2) *The blockage of a coronary artery by the accumulation of material in the wall of the*

13

artery (atheroma).

The usually smooth interior walls of the arteries become clogged with material. This development is accelerated in people who have high blood pressure. The inside of the artery grows lumpy and rough and restricts the flow of blood. Eventually enough material accumulates that the blood flow is completely halted. This seldom develops as the sole cause of a heart attack, however. More often the coronary artery is only partially closed by the build-up of fatty material. Then, other developments contribute to the attack as well. Most commonly it is the following two mechanisms, described below, which are involved.

3) *The blockage of an artery by a platelet plug.*

Platelets usually move along with the flow of blood. If, however, the blood vessel is damaged, the platelets tend to stick to the damaged area, creating a tight plug, which prevents the flow of blood. If a coronary artery becomes partially blocked by fatty material (as described in number 2 above), then there is a risk of platelets collecting very rapidly at a site and completely closing off the vessel, causing a heart attack.

14

4) *A spasm of the artery's wall causing block-age.*

Every arterial wall contains muscle, which is capable of contracting strongly if exposed to a very strong shock. There are many cases of major arteries being cut, yet not bleeding. The laceration stimulated muscle contraction which shut off the artery. It is possible, then, that an extraordinarily strong muscle contraction can indeed, block the artery completely, causing a heart attack. Scientists believe that stress triggers the heart to release chemicals which cause a spasm. The spasm reduces the oxygen supply.

Until relatively recently, medical professionals considered this a rare cause of heart attacks. With the advantages of new techniques and equipment, specialists are discovering, it is more common than they thought. Some think in fact, it may be the main cause of heart attacks. If this is, indeed, the case, it may mean that the damage caused by a heart attack may be reversible for up to several hours after the attack. If the spasm can be relieved and the blood can begin flowing again, permanent damage may be avoided.

15

Other Causes of Chest Pain

Whenever you feel a discomfort in your chest, your first instinct is to think its your heart. It's a common reaction, regardless of your age or state of health.

There are, however, many reasons for chest pain other than angina or a heart attack. Pain in this area may be caused by the lungs, the esophagus, or the abdomen. A virus, fungus or mold may also be a cause. Other causes include drinking cold liquids, or swallowing air while eating, talking or chewing gum.

In teenagers, an inflammation from a stretched ligament or minor problems in the bones and cartilage of the chest wall may be the reason for the pain. This can occur by bending forward, stretching, or reaching for an object as well as merely turning over in bed.

If you experience prolonged pain in your chest, it is best to visit a physician. Only your doctor can make an accurate diagnosis.

The following are brief descriptions of

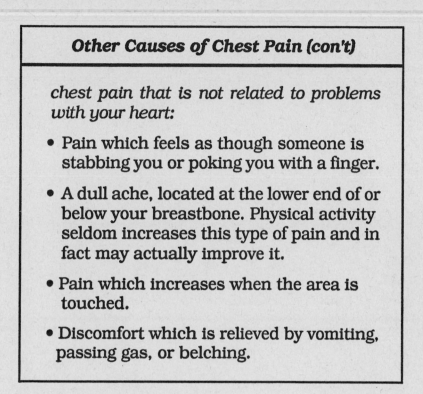

> ### *Other Causes of Chest Pain (con't)*
>
> *chest pain that is not related to problems with your heart:*
>
> - Pain which feels as though someone is stabbing you or poking you with a finger.
>
> - A dull ache, located at the lower end of or below your breastbone. Physical activity seldom increases this type of pain and in fact may actually improve it.
>
> - Pain which increases when the area is touched.
>
> - Discomfort which is relieved by vomiting, passing gas, or belching.

Technology to the Rescue

Back in 1912, when a Chicago banker suffered the first recorded heart attack, there was nothing physicians could do for him. Today, however, thanks to rapidly expanding technology there is help, both in terms of surgery and modern drugs.

Almost 20 years ago, bypass surgery was in its infancy. It wasn't even called that, but was referred to as "open heart" surgery. Very few people underwent it, not only because of the financial cost, but also because of the danger involved in this still new surgery.

Today it has become a routine procedure, with more than 170, 000 bypass operations being performed yearly in this country. Blood vessels are taken from a location of the body, for example the thigh, and are grafted into the diseased coronary artery. In this way, the blood is "re-routed" around the obstruction.

While it is used commonly, bypass surgery is still a traumatic operation to the patient, authorities explain, because the chest must remain open for several hours.

Even more advanced techniques may make the bypass operation obsolete, though. Balloon angioplasty is becoming an increasingly common operation since its inception nearly a decade ago. Its proper medical name is *Percutaneous Transluminal Coronary Angioplasty.*

The procedure involves inserting a catheter, or a thin flexible tube, into an artery through a small skin incision (percutaneously), usually in the groin, thigh or elbow area. The catheter is then threaded along the inside of the vessel (transluminally) to the area which is blocked.

The hollow catheter is only about 2 millimeters—1/12 of an inch—in diameter, Once the tube reaches the blockage, a tiny sausage-shaped balloon, located at the end of the catheter, is inflated with fluid, which causes distension of the artery (angioplasty) as well as a compression of the plaque against the artery wall.

The balloon is left inflated for several seconds and then is deflated. The procedure is repeated three times, with the pressure of the balloon being increased with each succeeding inflation.

The balloon is about two centimeters long-4/5 of a inch— when inflated and has a diameter of about two millimeters, 1/12 of an inch.

Balloon surgery is successful on about 80 percent of the patients and nearly 85 percent of these are healthy three years after the procedure.

The technique, however, has certain limits. It cannot compress arterial blockages that have been hardened through natural calcification, nor can it always clear total occlusions of the coronary arteries.

Laser Angioplasty

That's why laser angioplasty is so exciting. It was first used in 1983 by an America medical team working in Toulouse, France. This procedure also works on about 80 percent of the patients.

In this technique, laser energy vaporizes blood clots and plaque. The blockages are transformed into vapors and hydrocarbon molecules which are then dissolved in the bloodstream. It is, therefore, more effective than balloon angioplasty, which only compresses the fatty deposits. Lasers also have no trouble in cleaning the calcified deposits off arteries, something the balloon procedure cannot do.

Currently, Dr. James Forrester of Cedars-Sinai Medical Center in West Los Angeles is experimenting with a "cool" laser. This beam of concentrated light, which can remove a match's sulfur coating without igniting it, has already opened the arteries in more than 10 patients.

The laser energy is delivered through a flexible glass fiber optic tube, in the same fashion as is done in the balloon angioplasty. Dr. Forrester believes it will soon replace the invasive surgery in the treatment of leg arteries. "It's a major advance in the treatment of vascular disease because basically, you're eliminating the need for surgery," he said.

But it will be several years before it will be able to clear the smaller coronary arteries.The beating of the heart makes is difficult to aim the laser without running the risk of piercing a coronary artery wall.

Other Symptoms of Arterial Disease

The following is a list of symptoms also associated with arterial disease. Many of these one might *normally* relate to problems with the cardiovascular system. These signals, however, could be especially dangerous if you are over 30 years of age. Consult your physician if you experience any of them.

1) Frequent unexplained swelling of the ankles.

2) Memory loss and lapses into confusion.

3) Feeling of weakness—either generally or to a specific limb.

4) Fainting or blacking out for no apparent cause.

5) An ulceration on the ankle or foot which does not heal.

6) A white arc in the iris of the eye.

7) *Ringing in the ears*, or sudden partial deafness.

8) Sensation of vertigo.

Other Symptoms of Arterial Disease (con't)

9) A persistent coldness, numbness, tingling burning in the toes or feet.

10) Shortness of breath severe enough to make fast walking difficult.

11) Numbness in arms or legs.

Coronary Artery Disease

Coronary artery disease is the most serious—and most common—form of organic heart disease. The coronary arteries supply blood to the heart and have narrow central openings—called *lumens*—for blood flow. The widest of the lumens is about the *circumference of a small pea.* One can see how vital it is to keep these *lumens* free of atherosclerotic plaque. Should plaque begin to form and reduce the supply of blood to the heart, it may produce pain. The pain may not be felt directly on the heart, but it might be transmitted by nerve fibers to other parts of the body, such as the arms, neck or cheek.

Those afflicted with coronary artery

Coronary Artery Disease (con't)

damage may show one or more of the following symptoms:

1) *Heart Attack.* This may occur as a **first** outward sign of damage. The majority of heart attacks happen before a person actually reaches the hospital. Most are due to acute *arrhythmias.* Careful examination of thousands of heart attack victims showed that the average person waits four to five hours after experiencing pain before seeking help. Some people actually wait *days* as the symptoms increase in severity before they take action. It is estimated that nearly 150,000 people die each year because of delaying or refusing to seek medical attention.

2) *Congestive Heart Failure.* A series of symptoms, it includes the swelling of the lungs, heart murmurs and in some instances, ventricular *aneurysm*—the bulging out of the walls of the vein.

3) *Cardiac Arrhythmia.* An off-beat or ill-timed pumping of the heart, caused either by disorder of the impulse information or a problem with conduction from

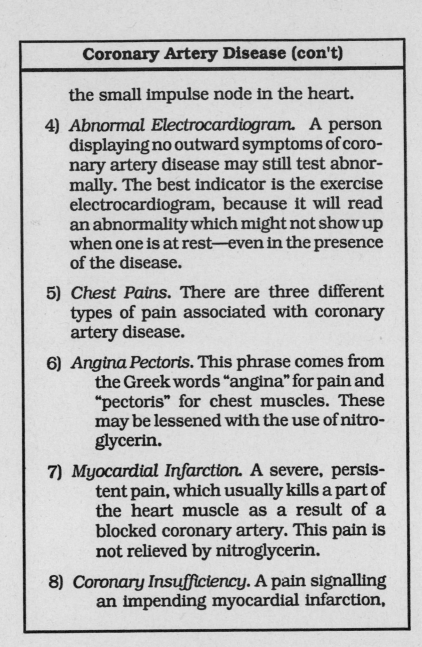

Coronary Artery Disease (con't)

the small impulse node in the heart.

4) *Abnormal Electrocardiogram.* A person displaying no outward symptoms of coronary artery disease may still test abnormally. The best indicator is the exercise electrocardiogram, because it will read an abnormality which might not show up when one is at rest—even in the presence of the disease.

5) *Chest Pains.* There are three different types of pain associated with coronary artery disease.

6) *Angina Pectoris.* This phrase comes from the Greek words "angina" for pain and "pectoris" for chest muscles. These may be lessened with the use of nitroglycerin.

7) *Myocardial Infarction.* A severe, persistent pain, which usually kills a part of the heart muscle as a result of a blocked coronary artery. This pain is not relieved by nitroglycerin.

8) *Coronary Insufficiency.* A pain signalling an impending myocardial infarction,

---

Coronary Artery Disease (con't)
but not yet associated with the death of the heart muscle. It includes inter-mediate syndromes which last longer than angina pectoris.

Myocarditis: Inflammation of the Heart

Myocarditis is an inflammation of the heart following a major viral infection. According to Dr. Walter H. Abelman, professor of medicine at Harvard University School of Medicine, this condition strikes between one and five percent of those who develop an infection The inflammation may be contained to a small area of the heart or it may cover a larger portion, Dr. Abelman noted.

It usually strikes people who refuse to rest properly while recovering from a viral attack which has been accompanied by a fever, the doctor explained.

The small area of inflammation can easily spread throughout the heart and possibly lead to irregular heart rhythm or heart failure.

It may also be caused by bacterial infections, radiation treatment for breast or lung cancer or chronic alcoholism.

Symptoms include difficulty in breathing, fatigue, palpitation, and fever. Occasionally, myocarditis may produce a mild continuous pressure or soreness in the chest.

If you believe you may have an inflammation of the heart, see your doctor immediately. Careful monitoring of the condition is required.

Smoking and The Heart

According to the medical community, the single most important step you can take in increasing your heart health is to stop smoking.

Even if you are following every suggestion in this book and those your doctor has outlined, your heart is gaining nothing if you still smoke. Medical researchers now know that cigarette smoking cancels out any other benefits to the heart. It will also have a negative effect on maintaining a healthy cholesterol level.

But, you say, you've tried and can't. Don't get discouraged. There are a lot of methods. If you can't go it alone, call your local lung association, they may know of some support groups. They may also know of successful ways others have kicked the habit. Below is the address for the national headquarters of the American Lung Association. They can refer you to the nearest branch.

American Lung Association
1740 Broadway
New York City, New York 10019

Chapter 2

The Healthy Road To A Normal Cholesterol Level

What causes this plaque on the arteries' walls which can do so much damage? In a word, cholesterol. It's a word we're all familiar with, if not through our family doctor, then through television advertising. Cholesterol is also a scary word for many people because it is a substance which contributes directly to heart disease. Elevated levels of cholesterol have been shown to increase significantly your chance's of developing atherosclerosis, or hardening of the arteries.

Medical authorities now believe that atherosclerosis is due to a disturbance of fat metabolism. Individuals whose blood demonstrates low levels of fatty substances—such as neutral fat, fatty acids, cholesterol, cholesterol esters and lipoproteins—also reveal a low incidence of atherosclerosis. And, those people who possess high levels of those fatty substances are more likely to develop hardening of the arteries.

27

Cholesterol is one of those fatty substances, but is is not a fat, even though its large molecule composition gives it some of the physical properties of fat.

It is, in fact, a necessary serum substance. Too much, we have all heard, can be dangerous to our health, however, too little can be just as dangerous.

The most widely known determination for the presence of atherosclerosis is the measurement of blood cholesterol. In the average American, this level varies from 180 mg to 200 mg per 100 cubic centimeters of blood. Those who register a higher blood cholesterol number—anywhere from 300 to 500 mg—also possess a higher incidence of atherosclerotic heart attacks than the general population, according to statistics.

Test Results Vary

The test, however, is subject to more errors and variations than almost any other laboratory procedure. One's emotional state, for example can cause a higher reading. Fear, depression, and anxiety may raise the level to twice its normal amount. It merely takes the fear of being poked with a needle it has been shown for some people to record higher readings.

Recently, another variation in test results has been discovered. According to Dr. Phillip Greenland of the University of Rochester (New York) School of Medicine and Dentistry, blood samples taken from the finger are consistently higher than samples taken from a vein.

From these findings, he concludes that about 10 percent of the people tested through the finger-prick method are sent for treatment on the basis of false high readings.

"This could result in added psychological stress (for the individual) and added cost in getting the answer straightened out," Dr. Greenland observed.

It might be a wise idea, if you have your cholesterol level checked by the finger-pricked method to ask for another test, with the blood being drawn from the vein this time.

Dr. Greenland also observed that cholesterol levels register higher during the winter months. He credits this to a "hibernation response" of the body.

Your Cholesterol Level

The National Institute of Health developed the following simple guidelines for reading cholesterol levels. These are general recommendations only. For specific factors related to your personal medical history, consult your physician. If you don't know your cholesterol level, your doctor can test you.

Blood Cholesterol Level
National Institute of Health Recommendations

Below 200—Desirable
To maintain this health level monitor your daily consumption of saturated fats.

200—239—Borderline
Restrict fats and saturated fats in your diet. Monitor your cholesterol level periodically.

200—239
Stringent dietary guidelines and/or medication may be required. Consult your physician for medical treatment.

240 and above—High
Medication and strict dietary guidelines may be required. Consult your physician for treatment and for a review of personal risk factors as outlined above.

The Benefits of Cholesterol

Television advertising beseeches us to reduce the amount of cholesterol in our diet. But the ads fail to mention that our bodies also produce cholesterol—and that it performs many vital functions. Too much cholesterol, medical authorities now say, is unhealthy. But, too little, also places the body in danger. Below are listed just some of the functions this much-maligned substance performs:

1) Forms nerve tissues.

2) Protects red blood cells.

3) Forms the main substance of cell walls.

4) Aids in the production of adrenal hormones.

5) Is the starting material for sex hormones.

6) Aids in the formation of bile acids, needed to properly assimilate fat.

The Good Guys Versus The Bad Guys

Cholesterol is a *lipid* produced in the liver from other food products at a rate of approximately one gram per day in the average adult male. When cholesterol combines with protein and *triglycerides*, also called neutral fats, the trio produces a *lipoprotein.*

31

Large particle lipoproteins are also referred to as *low density lipoproteins*—or LDL. They contain about 75 percent cholesterol. When blood cholesterol levels are tested, it is the LDL level which is being counted.

A second type of lipoprotein is formed from the combination of liver cholesterol and food protein. Called *high density lipoproteins*—or HDL—these substances are only now being identified as "the good guys." HDL apparently act as scavengers, actually clearing the body of cholesterol and then taking it to the liver for elimination.

Double Testing

The testing for LDL alone in your blood, therefore, might not be as effective as once thought. Doctors should consider performing tests to determine the amount of HDL as well. This provides more complete information about the status of your health.

For example, a reading of 300 mg is considered high, but in conjunction with an HDL value of more than 50 the risk of cardiovascular disease is markedly reduced. There are enough HDL to control the LDL.

On the other hand, a cholesterol test result of 225 is considered normal to borderline, depending upon the existence of other risk factors. If there exists a HDL value lower than 50, though, then there is cause for concern.

Women of childbearing years possess extra protection from LDL. Because of the production of female hormones, greater amounts of HDL and lesser amounts of LDL are produced. This is why the incidence of heart disease for women is lower. One note of caution, if you think you're completely free because you are female: In the past several years, the heart disease rate for women under 45 has increased by 11 percent. Some experts believe this is due to more women in high-pressure occupations.

**The Smokers' Cholesterol Level—
And Their Children's**

Doctors have long put those who smoke cigarettes at a higher risk for heart disease, because smoking hastens the development of hardening of the arteries. Up until recently, doctors weren't sure the reason why cigarettes did that. Now they are beginning to understand the process.

Research performed by Japanese scientists at Kyoto University indicates that cigarette smoke can change the low density lipoproteins—the "bad" cholesterol—so it is even more effective at sticking to the arteries and forming plaque.

Masayuki Yokodi, writing in the April 1988 *Proceedings of the National Academy of Sciences*, noted that the research involved animals, not humans. But, he explained, if the similar LDL modification can be found in humans (and there's little reason to doubt otherwise), then, it would "explain the increased incidence of atherosclerosis and coronary heart disease in smokers," he said.

The researchers noted modification of two LDL activities. The low density lipoprotein were "gobbled up" more readily by the macrophages, scavenger cells which help to convert the LDL to plaque. The second change was the increase in conversion to plaque. The smoke-treated LDL was converted 12.5 times faster than normal.

This research may also explain a new finding that boys with parents who smoke have a higher cholesterol level than boys from non-smoking families.

A research team from the Medical College of Virginia in Richmond, measured the levels of high density lipoprotein (HDL)—the cholesterol carrying agents which protect us from atherosclerosis—of 182 boys aged twelve. Forty one of the boys had a least one parent who smoked. The 141 live in non-smoking families. Those sons whose parents smoked had a 10 percent lower level of HDL.

Dr. William B. Moskowitz, who led the research, believes that the low HDL will eventually lead to a cholesterol build up in these children.

Girls did not show any change in cholesterol level, Dr. Moskowitz commented.

Phospholipids Join the Fight

Another vital part of lipoproteins are *phospholipids*—fat molecules which contain phosphorus. As a component of HDL, phospholipids prevent fat particles from attaching themselves to the arterial wall.

Similarly, the more phospholipids in LDL, the more favorable are a person's chances against developing cardiovascular disease.

A well-balanced diet provides an adequate amount of phosphorus for their formation. One should not think of cholesterol and phospholipids as separate substances, rather they are both very important components of lipoproteins.

Phosphorus, moreover, is vital to the body in other ways. It is an essential part of every tissue and cell in the body, even though nearly 90 percent of the trace mineral is found in the skeletal system.

An average of 0.88 grams daily has been determined to be needed for the maintenance of nutritional balance. The richest phosphorus containing supplement is lecithin. The Dr. Rinse Formula, discussed in Chapter Four, contains a good deal of lecithin.

Phosphorus is also found in body fluids along with magnesium, sodium potassium and calcium. There exists a rather delicate balance among these which influences the flexibility of the body's arterial walls as well as the elasticity and irritability of the muscles and nerves.

To illustrate just how vital these elements are to the working of the heart, consider this: The heart muscle's normal natural beating may be maintained for several hours after it is removed from the body. It is dependent, though, upon receiving a supply of artificial circulation of blood, lymph or a special water solution. With this technique it was discovered that the contractions and relations depend upon a balance of inorganic salts, which include phosphorus.

Garlic and Cholesterol

In addition to sound eating habits, there are natural ways to help reverse high cholesterol levels, some of which are quite easy to implement. *Garlic* is one of these all-natural methods. It is able to break down accumulated plaque which has formed inside the arteries.

The active ingredient responsible for this action is *allicin*, a sulfur-containing compound. The body transforms this into a substance which initiates a powerful internal "scrubbing" action which reduces the lipid levels in the blood-stream and the liver.

All you need to do is eat one or two cloves of garlic daily. George H. had a high cholesterol level. His doctor told him to modify his diet, but George explained he wasn't sure he could. The doctor, then, carefully outlined why it was vital that he try to change his eating habit. The physician also suggested to eat a clove of garlic daily.

At first, George thought his physician was kidding him but soon realized the doctor was very serious. The recommendation posed no problem, since George loved garlic. In fact, some days George would eat up to four cloves—usually two after lunch and another two after supper.

Within three weeks, his cholesterol level had

37

dropped considerably.

Eating garlic daily isn't always possible—or socially desirable. But there are plenty of garlic capsules on the market, which contain the powerful natural ingredients of garlic. One of the best found is *Garlimed,* by *Biowell,*which is made from an old Bulgarian formula. See the back of book for source of supply.

Pectin Lowers Cholesterol

Remember the old saying "an apple a day keeps the doctor away?" It has a lot of truth in it. Apples contain pectin, a water soluble substance that may be able to balance the ratio of HDL and LDL in your blood, and increase the level of good cholesterol in your blood.

Pectin is converted to an acid that combines with cholesterol tryglycerides and wastes to form an insoluble salt which is eliminated by the body.

The best way to consume apples for their pectin is with the skin, because this is where the concentration is the highest.

One medium sized apple contains approximately two grams of pectin. Your body needs about 10 grams a day to reduce the levels of LDL in your blood.

Don't worry, you don't have to eat five apples a day "to keep the doctor away." A variety of foods also contain pectin, including pineapples, raspberries, avocados, tomatoes, grapes, peaches, cherries and bananas.

Calcium's Role in Lowering Cholesterol

Recent research indicates that the mineral, *calcium,* which we most closely associate with strong, healthy bones, may also have the ability to lower serum cholesterol.

According to research conducted by Anthony A. Albanese, Ph.D., and several of his colleagues, calcium was responsible for lowering the cholesterol level of a group of women, between the ages of 53 and 88. These women took 750 mg of calcium daily, as well as Vitamin D to enhance the mineral's absorption.

A control group taking a placebo received no benefits. The doctors hope that calcium "may prove to be a meaningful therapeutic action in the management of cardiovascular diseases."

Similar results were found in another test, which involved men and women between the ages of 26 and 61. It was conducted by Alan I. Fleischman, Ph.D. and M.L. Biernbaum, M.D. of the

Atherosclerosis Research group at St. Vincent's Hospital in Montclair, New Jersey.

All of the subjects in the group had high levels of cholesterol and other fats circulating in their blood. Three of the subjects had previously suffered heart attacks and three had experienced angina pains.

They took 2,000 mg of calcium divided into four daily doses for one year. Their serum cholesterol level fell an average of 24 percent. The researchers reported no adverse side effects with that large of calcium intake.

Calcium appears to act as a cholesterol normalizer, the researchers say. It worked best on people with especially high initial cholesterol readings, while bringing a moderate reduction in those with only slightly elevated levels. And, most significantly, for those who had normal cholesterol levels, the calcium supplements produced no change.

Alfalfa: A Natural Way to Lower Cholesterol

As a method of lowering cholesterol, alfalfa works in the intestinal tract, where it binds with cholesterol and carries it out of the system, before it can be absorbed by the body, medical specialists explain.

Nutritionists recommend a daily salad which includes lots of alfalfa sprouts. If that isn't possible, they suggest alfalfa tablets. Four taken before each of the three meals of the day is advised. It is important that the tablets are taken before you eat, so that hey have the opportunity to combine with the dietary cholesterol.

Vitamin E

Vitamin E is gaining increasing respect from scientists, especially when it comes to lowering the cholesterol levels.

A team of physicians from the Wood Veterans Administration Medical Center in Milwaukee, Wisc., tested the effects of this vitamin on 43 people. They gave each person 800 I.U. (International Units) of Vitamin E daily for a period of one month. Results of the test clearly showed that some of the people had higher HDL levels—the "good" cholesterol which escorts the LDL out of the body. Curiously, the levels were raised only in those who initially had low HDL readings.

Similar results were found by William J. Herman, M.D.,. a pathologist in Houston, Texas. He discovered that Vitamin E was most effective on people who had low HDL levels, who were younger than 35 years and who were no more than 10

41

percent over their ideal weight.

Magnesium

Dr. Paavo Airola, the world famous nutritionist, recommends those at risk of developing hardening of the arteries take 400 mg of magnesium daily.

It is an excellent preventative measure to ensure a low cholesterol count as well as a healthy heart. Remember, it is one of the components of the body fluid which is essential for the heart's continuous healthy beating. It is also essential in regulating the enzyme production which helps keep atherosclerosis in check.

Moreover, a shortage of magnesium cannot only cause calcification of the arteries, but it can also produce irregular heart beats.

An excellent product found which combines the benefits of Vitamin E and magnesium is *Cardio-san*™ , by *Biowell*. This all-natural supplement will help you keep your cholesterol count in check and ensure your heart receives the benefits of the natural ingredients of the formula.

Calcium Pectate

Carrots have been touted lately to be a great source of beta carotene, which many specialists say is a natural protection from cancer, especially the lung. Now there's more reason than ever to munch on a couple carrots. Research is showing that this root may also lower your cholesterol.

Carrots are also an excellent source of *calcium pectate*, a type of fiber which makes them an especially potent cholesterol-fighting weapon, according to two researchers at the U.S. Department of Agriculture's Eastern Regional Research Center in Philadelphia.

The center's Peter Hoagland, Ph.D. and Philip Pfeiffer, Ph.D. explain that calcium pectate is found in the cell walls of the carrot. It binds with bile acids which are made from cholesterol and other substances in the liver. When this occurs, the body doesn't need to make its own cholesterol to increase the supply.

Dr. Hoagland says that by eating two medium sized carrots daily, you may be able to lower your cholesterol level by 10 or even 20 percent.

Calcium pectate is also found in cabbage and onions. One cup chopped onions or cabbage daily should provide the same effects, he observed.

Oat Bran

Oatmeal was once the food you ate grudgingly because your mother said it was good for you. She was right—it is good for you. And scientists are only now confirming how effective oat bran is at lowering cholesterol levels.

Eating oatmeal daily has been shown to lower the low density lipoproteins (LDL) by nearly 25 percent. Current research seems to show that the longer you continue to eat the food—the lower your cholesterol level will fall.

And you don't have to eat a lot of it. About one and a half to three ounces of oat bran daily will do the trick.

"It's great stuff," Dr. James Anderson of the University of Kentucky at Lexington remarked. He is the researcher who first discovered the cholesterol-reducing properties of this food nearly a decade ago.

Scientists credit oat bran's high content of soluble fiber for its health benefits. This is why oat bran works more effectively than wheat bran at lowering cholesterol levels. Wheat bran contains only 3.3 grams of soluble fiber per 100 grams, while oat bran contains 14 grams.

Oat bran is available in just about every health

food store as well as most grocery stores. And while you can eat it as a hot cereal there are also many ways to add oat bran into your diet. Muffins are an ideal food, when homemade with the bran. Homemade breads and rolls are other good sources.

Suggested Dietary Guidelines
For Low Cholesterol

The following are suggestions to help you lower your intake of saturated fats, cholesterol, and salt. This will contribute greatly to lowering your chances of developing hardening of the arteries.

* Reduce by one-half your consumption of fatty meats—beef, lamb, bacon, spare ribs, sausage and lunch meats. Instead, eat fish, poultry and foods rich in complex carbohydrates.

* Trim the fat off the few meats you do eat. *Broil* or *roast* the meat instead of frying it. *Avoid* organ meats, such as liver and brains.

* Avoid fast food, processed or convenience foods, as well as commercial baked goods.

* Eliminate or drastically reduce your intake of high salt foods, such as bacon, ham, sausage, frankfurters, lunch meats, salted nuts and salted snack foods, such as potato chips, french fries, corn chips, etc.

Suggested Dietary Guidelines
For Low Cholesterol (con't)

* Gradually cut down your use of salt at the dinner table and replace it with herbs. Cut your use of salt in cooking by two-thirds. Use salt substitutes if you feel you still need salt. Be creative in cooking with herbs, lemon, spices and vinegar made from apples or red wine.

* Increase your intake of whole fruits and vegetables, lightly milled and whole grains, such as whole wheat bread, cracked wheat, rolled oats, brown rice, rye and millet.

* Switch from hard margarine to *unsalted butter*. Instead of lard or shortening use unhydrogenated vegetable oil. Whenever possible, use cold-pressed, *unrefined* flaxseed oil, such as *C-Leinomed*.

* Reduce by one-half your weekly servings of whole milk, ice cream, cheese (except for the low-fat varieties).

* Switch from ice cream to ice milk, from whole milk to non-fat milk and from regular to non-fat yogurt.

The Importance of Dietary Fats

The American Heart Association has published research showing that the American diet is both excessively high in the wrong kinds of fats and deficient in the right kinds. Health experts world-wide have documented the problems arising as a result of consuming too much of the wrong type of fat.

The organization has issued dietary guidelines which strongly suggest that we can reduce our risk of developing heart disease (as well as other degen-erative diseases) simply by trimming no less than 10 percent of the fat from our daily menus.

On the surface of it, this seems to be an easy guideline to observe. It's really not difficult for the family cook to skim off the fat that rises to the top of the pot when making soups, stews, and gravies. Fish with lemon and herbs is even more delicious than a greasy hamburger, and a lot healthier. Every supermarket in the country carries well-known and heavily-advertised name brands of margarines and vegetable oils that proudly claim to be *free* of the saturated fats that promote harm-ful blood cholesterol levels. Every refrigerator case in every supermarket holds a vast selection of low-fat dairy products. Even salad dressings and may-onnaises especially processed to be low in fat, are now readily available.

But—and *it's a big but*—just how healthy are these commercially processed fats and oils? Be-cause medical researchers and scientists all over the world have found that the excessive consump-

47

tion of dietary fats can be dangerous to our health, we decided to do some serious in-depth digging to find out the *real* story behind the brief dietary guidelines suggesting a reduction in fats which have been issued in recent years.

THE OIL PROCESSING INDUSTRY

The industry as we know it has been growing by leaps and bounds for over fifty years. However, medical detectives and scientists have made some startling discoveries in the past two decades about the way fat metabolism works (or doesn't work) in the body. Perhaps if we had known fifty years ago what we know now about the ways in which chemically altered fats lead to a host of degenerative diseases, the government might have taken a different position on these products. According to reliable sources, the methods used by the commercial oil industry to manufacture dietary fats are subject to "periodic" review and re-evaluation by the Food & Drug Administration. In light of the growing masses of clinical research about the harmful effects of excessive fat intake, perhaps it's time to call for the FDA to exercise their prerogatives and do a thorough review of industry manufacturing methods in order to update their records.

In the industrialized societies, the increased incidence of the degenerative diseases (cancer, cardiovascular disease, diabetes, multiple sclerosis, liver and kidney problems) have paralleled the increased consumption of unnatural chemically altered fats. That may be a bold statement, but it's easily documented. A whopping 57 percent of our dietary fat consumption now comes from commercially processed fats and oils, such as margarine, shortening, salad and cooking oils. At the turn of the century, cancer claimed the life of one person in every thirty, but today it kills one in five. One hundred years ago, heart disease took one person in every seven. The cardiovascular toll is now one person in every two.

Destructive "Industrial Strength" Fats

You may find it hard to believe what the commercial oil industry does with some perfectly natural seeds before you find the finished products (margarine, cooking and salad oils, shortening) on the shelves of your neighborhood grocery stores. Here's what happens during the processing methods:

"COLD-PRESSED"—After the seeds are cleaned, they are mechanically crushed and subjected to fierce temperature (the average is around 248 degrees F.) in order to break down the cell walls, thereby making the extraction of the oil easier.

49

Because the vital live enzymes cannot survive temperatures much over 100 degrees F., it's already too late to save the enzymes, but we're just beginning. Next, the unappetizing dead mash of cooked seeds is forced through a giant press that works very much like an old-fashioned kitchen meat grinder. The difference is that this press exerts tremendous pressure (up to several tons per square inch). As the screw inexorably turns, the seeds are crushed and forced against the press head. This friction generates more heat (up to 203 degrees F.). This combination of friction-generated heat and press-crushing forces the seed to give up its oil.

If the processing stops here, these oils are allowed to be sold (usually in health-food stores at a premium price) as "cold-pressed," "natural," "crude," or "unrefined." Most authorities agree that the temperatures generated in the processing are high enough to cause deterioration of the essential fatty acids. As hard as it may be to believe, these "cold-pressed" oils are the highest quality currently from U.S. manufacturers.

"UNREFINED OIL"—Another favored method of extraction consists of using a chemical solvent to leach the oil from seeds. After being crushed and cooked, the seeds are then mechanically ground and processed with a chemical solvent at temperatures of up to 149 degrees F. (One popular solvent is hexane, manufactured from petroleum). You should know that the solvent is reclaimed after batches of seeds have been processed and is re-used many times. Oils extracted with chemicals are unavoidably tainted with traces of these chemicals. Very often, chemically extracted oils are mixed with "cold-pressed" oils. These oils find their way to stores and are marketed as "unrefined oils."

You Asked For It

Consumers have been brain-washed into believing that their salad and cooking oils should be clear, free-occurring at any temperature, odorless, and tasteless. Without commercial processing, natural oils offer the delicate taste characteristic of the seeds from which they came. They range in color from a pale yellow to gold to amber to almost red. Their different aromas are as distinctive as their different tastes. If you put them in the refrigerator, they become cloudy and their viscosity changes. In other words, they become somewhat heavier and thicker.

THE REFINING PROCESS—The first step in refining the oil, called degumming, is to remove most of the remaining phosphatides, essential for life. Lecithin (an important unsaturated fatty acid) is taken out. All the complex carbohydrates, some elements similar to proteins, and the gums are removed. The chlorophyll, calcium, magnesium, iron, and copper (health-promoting minerals) are also refined out.

Second, some caustic corrosive chemicals, such as sodium hydroxide (better known as Draino), or a mixture of sodium hydroxide and sodium carbonate, are dumped into the oil. The nasty mess is then mechanically agitated at a temperature of approximately 167 degrees F. The remaining free fatty acids combine with the caustic chemicals to form easily removed "soaps." Just about all that's left of the remaining minerals, protein-like elements, and phospholipids (fats with phosphorous and nitrogen), are eliminated furring this stage of the "refining" process. But the oil may be yellowish or reddish in color, still hanging on to a little of its identity in the form of pigments.

The third step consists of bleaching out the natural pigments to provide you with that colorless oil you've been taught to expect. Beta-carotene (a documented cancer-preventive) and chlorophyll, along with the last traces of the fatty acids, are filtered out, usually with acid-based clays, at temperatures of up to 230 degrees F. The essential fatty acids still present are further chemically damaged and may form toxic peroxides.

Deodorizing is the fourth step in the refining process. You couldn't possibly recognize the seed source of the oil at this point. The delicate flavor and scent that Mother Nature puts into her seeds has been replaced by unappetizing chemical odors and tastes. Taking out the bad taste and smell is accomplished by the use of a steam distilling process at extremely high temperatures (up to 518 degrees F.) for a period lasting as long as an hour. Thankfully, the dangerous peroxides and toxins produced in the previous step are removed, along with some of the pesticide residue. But the deodorizing process also eliminates the Vitamin E. And, of immense concern to all of us, the essential fatty acids have been transformed into something completely foreign to the human body.

The oil must undergo yet another couple of steps before you buy it and take it home. Because the natural antioxidants Beta-Carotene and Vitamin E have been removed from the oil in the "refining process," synthetic chemical antioxidants are pumped in to lengthen the shelf life and a "defoamer" is also added. And, because some of us refrigerate our salad and cooking oils, it is usually subjected to a process known in the industry as "winterization." The oil is artificially cooled and filtered yet again to insure that it remains clear under refrigeration. (This is the "polyunsaturated" oil that is commonly added to commercial baby

53

formulas to provide "essential fatty acids.")

The end result is an oil that is clear, odorless, tasteless, and indistinguishable from any other oil manufactured in the same manner. Unless the label tells you, there's absolutely no way to tell what the original seed source might have been. With all the vitamins and minerals eliminated, and the essential fatty acid molecules chemically altered, that oil on your supermarket shelves is a highly questionable food item.

Adding Insult To Injury

THE HYDROGENATION PROCESS—Even if the industry started with a completely natural oil (and they don't, they start with a chemically altered one), the hydrogenation process destroys all nutritional value. Hydrogenating the oil consists of completely saturating all of the fatty acids with hydrogen. Hydrogenation is accomplished under pressure by using temperatures of up to 410 degrees F. in the company of a metal catalyst (nickel, platinum, copper) for as long as eight hours. Because the final product is a completely inert (dead) substance, it doesn't spoil and can be heated for (or in) cooking without becoming dangerously toxic. But it contains chemically altered bits of fatty acids, some of which may be harmful, and traces of the metal catalyst.

PARTIAL HYDROGENATION—By controlling the length of the hydrogenation process, a liquid oil can be transformed into a solid or semi-solid mass of fat. When the desired degree of hardness is attained, the hydrogenation process is stopped. Margarines and solid shortenings are manufactured with partially hydrogenated oils. Although logically you might not think so, *partially* hydrogenated products are actually more dangerous to your health than *fully* hydrogenated products. Here's why:

The molecules in the oil being bombarded with hydrogen become saturated (hydrogenated) erratically, leaving behind a proliferation of strangely altered substances when the process is halted. Many of these chemically alien elements are identified as being harmful because they interfere with the body's normal metabolism. Many others have not been scientifically researched and we just don't know what dangers they may pose when ingested.

MARGARINE—The Encyclopedia Britannica tells us that French chemist Hippolyte Mege-Mouries invented "artificial butter" back in 1869. Mege-Mouries won the prize offered by Napoleon, who wanted a cheap fat to feed his soldiers and sailors, with his combination of skim milk and suet (melted beef fat). Although this disagreeable early

55

butter substitute tasted just as awful as it sounds, it caught on. Mege-Mouries secured a patent for his process in the United States in 1873 and the industry as we know it today began.

As time passed, the animal fats used in the beginning gave way to imported vegetable fats, usually cottonseed, soybean, peanut, and corn oils, and the product became more palatable. The early manufacture of margarine was subject to strong restrictive legislation in the U.S. because both the butter producers and the nation's farmers feared for their livelihood. However, during the 1930's, U.S. farmers began supplying cottonseed and soybeans and the fledgling "artificial butter" industry was on its way. As recently as World War II, margarine was sold uncolored. The white block, looking like a brick of shortening, came with a packet of powdered yellow-orange dye which the housewife had to blend in, usually by squeezing it through the softened mass with her hands.

No matter what seed oil the margarine manufacturer starts with, and usually the cheapest source is used, the essential fatty acids present to start with are either destroyed or changed in the hydrogenation process into chemically altered substances. The essential fatty acids that remain fight with the carbon fatty acids and reduce the nutritional value of the essentials still further. Add to this the fact that the minerals and vitamins the body needs for efficient metabolism of fats, were "refined" out and you have a nearly indigestible fat.

A very efficient advertising campaign has led us to believe that margarine is good for us because it's made with polyunsaturated fats. We equate poly-unsaturated with good health because we know that the essential fatty acids are polyunsaturated. But what they don't tell us is that the polyunsaturated fats in margarine are not the essential fatty acids the body needs, but chemically-altered alien fats. It is true that margarine contains no cholesterol, but the presence of so many chemicals completely alien to the body cancels out that small advantage. Remember, there is a lot of evidence showing that these chemically altered fats are strongly implicated in the degenerative diseases.

HOW MUCH IS TOO MUCH?—A lot of very authoritative medical scientists hold the position that the body reacts adversely to even a smidgin of a chemically-altered alien substance. The cumulative effects of regularly consuming a diet high in these fats are devastating.

Studies show that hard margarines contain an average of over 30 percent chemically altered fatty acids. (Some brands register a whopping 60 percent.) Soft margarines (and diet margarines) contain an average of close to 20 percent chemically altered fatty acids. The measurable essential *fatty acids* present in margarines are virtually zero—less than 5 percent chemically-altered fatty acids.

Commercially made baked goods average nearly 35 percent chemically-altered fatty acids. Even that old standby, peanut butter, contains varying amounts of chemically-altered fatty acids. I hate to tell you about french fries (up to 40 percent) and potato chips (another 40 percent).

Is butter better than margarine? Well, it is certainly natural and tastes better. Unfortunately, of the 500 fatty acids which have been identified in butter, only a very small percentage are the essentials (linoleic acid 2%, linolenic acid, trace). Over 65 percent of butter's fatty acid content requires the same elements for metabolism as the essentials. If the non-essential fatty acids outnumber the essentials, it's easy to understand that the non-essentials will win the metabolic battle. Butter also contains a small (less than 5 percent) amount of chemically altered fatty acids. Unlike the chemically processed fats and oil discussed earlier, these altered fats are produced in the cow itself and are not a serious health risk.

Butter does contain about 1 gram of cholesterol in every pound. The average diet is sadly lacking in the elements (essential fatty acids, certain vitamins and minerals) needed to process cholesterol efficiently. The natural diet consumed by our ancestors had these elements in abundance.

Another drawback is that our modern-day butter also registers the presence of unwanted pesticides and antibiotics. The cows feed on grasses and grains that are pesticide-treated. Antibiotics are routinely given to the animals themselves and commercially manufactured feed is treated with antibiotics. The target is harmful disease-promoting bacteria, which are destroyed by the antibiotic treatment. But some friendly bacteria have developed resistance to the drugs. With good reason, researchers fear that the resistance factor can cross over to the dangerous bacteria, making them less susceptible to antibiotics.

In favor of butter, we must point out that it can be used in and for all types of cooking without breaking down into dangerous toxins. It is stable in the presence of light, heat, and oxygen, The relatively small percentage of naturally-occurring altered fatty acids is not a threat to health, but you can't depend on butter for your supply of essential fatty acids. Butter is easy to digest and the cholesterol content is not harmful, as long as your diet contains the elements necessary for the efficient metabolism of fat. However, even this natural dietary fat can create problems when consumed in excess. To sum it all up, butter is better for you, unless you're a glutton about it.

It's important to remember that fatty acids are essential to the entire body. It's therefore very important to seek out and incorporate good sources of the right kind of fatty acids into your daily diet. The following diagram illustrates the relationships of polyunsaturated dietary fatty acids and their influence on human diseases.

Presence of Polyunsaturated Fatty Acids in Various Oils and Their Influence on Human Diseases.

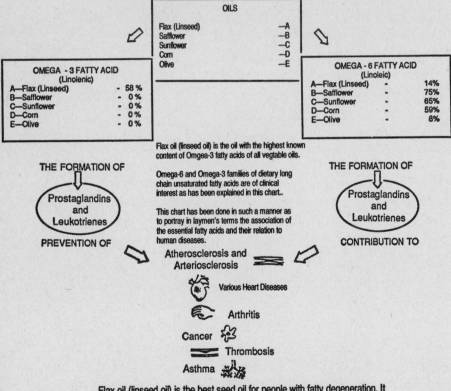

OILS

Flax (Linseed)	—A
Safflower	—B
Sunflower	—C
Corn	—D
Olive	—E

OMEGA - 3 FATTY ACID
(Linolenic)

A—Flax (Linseed)	- 58 %
B—Safflower	- 0%
C—Sunflower	- 0%
D—Corn	- 0%
E—Olive	- 0%

OMEGA - 6 FATTY ACID
(Linoleic)

A—Flax (Linseed)	- 14%
B—Safflower	- 75%
C—Sunflower	- 65%
D—Corn	- 59%
E—Olive	- 8%

Flax oil (linseed oil) is the oil with the highest known content of Omgea-3 fatty acids of all vegtable oils.

THE FORMATION OF

Prostaglandins and Leukotrienes

PREVENTION OF

Omega-6 and Omega-3 families of dietary long chain unsaturated fatty acids are of clinical interest as has been explained in this chart..

This chart has been done in such a manner as to portray in laymen's terms the association of the essential fatty acids and their relation to human diseases.

THE FORMATION OF

Prostaglandins and Leukotrienes

CONTRIBUTION TO

Atherosclerosis and Arteriosclerosis

Various Heart Diseases

Arthritis

Cancer

Thrombosis

Asthma

Flax oil (linseed oil) is the best seed oil for people with fatty degeneration. It disperses from our tissues deposits of the unsaturated fatty acids and cholesterol, which like to aggregate and make platelets sticky.

Flax oil (linseed oil) should be unrefined, fresh and when opened kept refrigerated for it to retain its full potency.

60

Fats Affect The Entire Body

The human body benefits greatly from essential fatty acids. And these fatty acids are of great concern for the person who is at risk, or already suffers from high cholesterol and other forms of heart disease.

When we compare a healthy heart with one that has experienced a heart attack, we find the diseased heart is burdened with an accumulation of fat.

The first visible symptom of many degenerative diseases is the separation of lipids from the surrounding tissue. Saturated, hydrogenated, chemically-hardened fats can actually act as chemical carcinogens within the body. Research indicates the trouble begins when the protein-bound fats, normally present as free-flowing lipids in a live organism, become separated from their protein carriers and end up as unhealthy deposits in various parts of the body.

FATS ARE IMPORTANT—Science has proven that fats play an important part in the functioning of the entire body. Fats (lipids) are vital for all growth processes, renewal of cells, brain and nerve functions, even for the sensory organs (eyes and ears), and for the body's adjustment to heat, cold, and quick temperature changes. Our energy re-

61

sources are based on lipid metabolism.

Each and every cell in the body is protectively covered with a sheath of fats. The cell body (plasma) is interlaced with little lipid veins, often called the "nerves of the cell." These lipid nerve-veins are the connection between the nucleus and the outer membrane. They influence the care and feeling of the cell and the process of normal cell division by the use of tiny electrical impulses. To function efficiently, cells require polyunsaturated live *electron-rich* lipids, present in abundance in *crude flax oil*. Polyunsaturated fats greedily absorb proteins and oxygen. It is a documented fact that many people suffer from an oxygen shortage simply because they are deficient in these oxygen-active lipids.

Lipids are only water-soluble and free-flowing when bound to protein, thus forming an electric counterpole to their protein carriers. This vitally important type of fat contains accumulated energy in its electron clouds. When high quality electron-rich fats are combined with proteins, the electrons are protected until the body requires energy. This energy source is fully and immediately available to the body on demand, as nature intended. These energy resources can be instantly mobilized and rushed into action as needed.

The presence of these important lipids can be

compared to the capital (money reserves) of a corporation. Any type of growth or activity, whether that of a corporation or the human body, requires an expenditure of capital (money or energy). In the body, any activity (physical or mental) or growth factor (during pregnancy or the normal growing period from infant to adult, for example) requires the presence of electron-rich fats bound to proteins. All the cells, muscle masses, brain, nerves, organs, and lifestreams (blood and lymph) of the body need these electrically-charged, highly-active lipids. The demands on these energy reserves are enormous. Every breath we take, every muscle we move, every time the heart beats—even the automatic process of renewal and division of every cell in the body—depends on this energy source.

Let's examine the benefits accruing to the heart from electrically-charged lipids. There is an immediate harmonious interaction with the heart when the spent venous blood receives a healthy dose of lipids from the lymphatic system immediately before entering the heart. Inside the heart, the venous blood and lipids are mixed, creating a measurable electric current which regulates the action of the heart and sends impulses to the entire circulatory system. This blood, now charged by the electron-rich lipids, then flows to the lungs where it is charged with oxygen and pumped through the left ventricle into the aortas of the body. The vital life-sustaining pumping action of the heart itself depends on the electrical charge created by the lipids.

THE IMPORTANT FOODS—Many of the foods we commonly eat are lacking in both essential fatty acids and essential amino acids. The essential amino acids (proteins) are present in abundance in cottage cheese, buttermilk, hard cheeses, whole wheat, fish, and lean meats. The essential fatty acids the body hungers for are found in rich supply in crude, unrefined flax oil, soy lecithin, egg yolks, and some vegetable oils. The problem, of course, with most commercially processed vegetable oils that stock the shelves of our supermarkets is that they are heated, refined, hydrogenated, and full of chemical preservatives. Because the essential fatty acids are particularly sensitive to heat and oxidation, margarines and processed vegetable oils no longer carry their content of essential fatty acids.

It is only when the body is well supplied with the essential fatty acids and essential amino acids in proper balance that the metabolic system can function as nature intends it to. In the presence of these vital elements, healthy oxygenated blood courses richly throughout the entire organism to benefit every cell. When the essential fatty acids bind with the essential amino acids, the offspring of this happy marriage are called "lipoproteins." Healthy people have an abundance of lipoproteins but it has been observed that diseased patients (including victims of cancer) have a much reduced level of lipoproteins in their blood, or none at all.

By comparing the body to a wood or coal burning stove, perhaps we can form an easily understood mental picture, albeit very simplified, of the workings of the body. Let's say that the stove has been overheated often, it has been fed the cheapest grade of coal, and its maintenance has been neglected for a long period of time. The body of the stove, the stovepipe, and the chimney become clogged with a dangerous residue that could flare into flames at any time, and which might very well burn down the house. We must clean away the deposits and feed the stove well-dried wood that burns cleanly without leaving a harmful residue.

The body which has been wrongly fed, poorly maintained, and neglected is in the same sad state as the abused stove. Harmful deposits and a residue of fats clog the inner workings of the body. By introducing the clean essential fatty acids present in *flax oil* and the superior high quality proteins (amino acids) present in cottage cheese, the body immediately goes to work to rid itself of the deposits inhibiting its normal functioning. By continuing to feed the body with these good natural nutrients, soon the body becomes healthy again as nature intended.

Needless to say, after the body has been efficiently cleansed and is free of harmful deposits, we're certainly not going to return to the same old suspect foods that caused the problem in the first place. In order to stay well, the experts say that good dietary habits must be followed rigorously for a lifetime.

EXAMINING CHEMICALLY-PROCESSED FATS—Many doctors preach against the use of what we they call "pseudo" fats. In order to extend the shelf life, to provide the market with a visually attractive assortment of liquid and artificially hardened fats (margarines) — in short, to make money, manufacturers use chemical processes that render their products harmful to the body. These fats may be market "polyunsaturated," but they are damaging to the body all the same.

The chemical processing of fats destroys the vital electron cloud, demonstrated in the foregoing material to be of immense importance to the functioning of every cell in the body. Once the electrons have been removed, these fats can no longer bind with oxygen and actually become an obstacle to the process of breathing. The heart rejects these fats and they end up as inorganic fatty deposits on the heart muscle itself. A diseased heart and its aortas clearly show deposits of these worthless, electrically dead lipids.

Chemically processed fats are not water-soluble when bound to protein. They end up blocking circulation, damaging heart action, inhibiting cell renewal, and impeding the free flow of blood and lymph fluids. The bio-electrical action in these areas slows down and may become completely paralyzed. The entire organism shows a measurable loss of the electrical energy which is replenished only by adding active lipids to the diet. These nutritional fats are truly vital for man.

In recent years, scientists have coined the term "fat intolerance" and deplore the damage done by fat degeneration. The body rejects chemically-processed fats because their composition has been changed so drastically from what nature intended that they are no longer able to fulfill their function in the organism, but instead cause untold damage to the body.

It is interesting to note that Russia outlawed the chemical saturation of fats for the purpose of causing them to harden artificially, as in the production of margarine, as long ago as 1902. Dr. Budwig explains that it is impossible to correct the damage done to lipids once they have been hardened into margarine just by adding linoleic acid. In order to obtain a high level of linoleic acid, the manufacturers put in a chemical combination of ethyl and methyl esters, not the pure natural oil.

67

Much research has documented the fact that this type of artificial linoleic acid does not combat the symptoms of an essential fatty acid deficiency in the body.

In direct contrast to the chemically-produced fatty acids, consider what happens when just a minute quantity (one microgram) of *flax oil* is introduced into the bloodstream of a heart patient. Because the natural fatty acids present in *crude flax oil* easily bind with oxygen and protein, the blood of the patient improves within four to six hours. The activity of these natural lipids in the blood stream can actually be microscopically observed.

Fat damage is apparent in the heart, the liver and the arteries. The source of this degenerative damage lies in faulty nutrition, in the intake of the wrong kinds of fats. These findings have been substantiated by cancer researchers from twenty-nine NATO countries. Surely, no health-care practitioner, no scientist, and no thinking person can continue to ignore these facts. The essential electronically-charged fats that are found in abundance in natural *flax oil* are crucially important to the health and functioning of the body.

Research is proving that the most favorable way to attack cholesterol and heart disease at their roots is by removing all "pseudo" fat from the diet and in their place introducing the true nutrition of the natural medicinal fats present in *unrefined flaxseed oil,* such as C-*Leinomed, by Biowell.* (See last page of book).

HIGH FAT CONSUMPTION—Statistics show that overall fat consumption is increasing. Research conducted with laboratory animals provides important insight into one of the metabolic disorders arising from the overconsumption of saturated fats. Lab animals fed a diet high in saturated fats greedily consume as much as five to six times as much food (including fats) as animals fed a normal diet. Even more important, this study showed that when the animals were fed natural fats from flaxseed, they consumed only about one-fifth of the fat and one-fifth of other foods in comparison with the group of animals fed saturated fats.

This experiment showed very graphically that "cheap" fats are actually very expensive, both in terms of cost and in terms of health. In an effort to ingest the essential fatty acids their bodies craved, the lab animals ate five times as much of the commercially processed fats as did the animals supplied with the electron-rich active natural fats. This may very well be the explanation of just why our overall fat consumption is increasing. After all, the human body is not so very different from the body of an animal bred for laboratory research.

The health and well-being of the organism depends entirely on the type of nutrition consumed. Research demonstrates that normal growth, healthy skin, glandular functions (liver, gall bladder, pancreas, stomach, intestines, prostate, lymph), are especially dependent on active fats. Glandular secretions are dependent on natural protein-reactive lipids. When chemically processed fats (protein and oxygen inactive) are consumed, there is a consequent inhibiting of all glandular activity within the system.

One of the first symptoms of faulty fat metabolism, easily observed by any of us, is a drying of the mucous membranes of the nose and mouth. The dried-out membranes, resulting in a sore, raspy voice, are caused when the glandular secretions are inhibited by the ingestion of chemically processed fats. Not so easily recognized, but just as harmful, is the drying effect exerted on the entire digestive and intestinal tract.

The Important Fats

Cholesterol is dissolved and held in suspension in a free-flowing liquid state in the blood in the presence of adequate essential fatty acids. Because the melting point of cholesterol is 300 de-

70

grees Fahrenheit, it is deposited on arterial walls as an insoluble substance at the normal body temperature of 98.6 degrees Fahrenheit.

With the fatty acid lecithin present, the melting point of cholesterol is reduced to 180 degrees Fahrenheit, which is much lower than previously, but still insoluble at body temperature. But when the essential fatty acids, linoleic and linolenic, as found in the flax oil, *C-Leinomed*, are insufficient supply, the melting point of cholesterol comes down to 32 degrees Fahrenheit, well below normal body temperature. In a liquid state, cholesterol cannot remain as harmful arterial plaque and does not promote the degenerative diseases.

FISH OIL—There's been a lot written lately about the omega-3 fatty acids *(eicosapentaenoic acid* [EPA] and *docosahexaenoic acid* [DHA] present in the arterial-cleansing fish oils. The fact that Eskimos and the Scandinavian peoples eat a lot of cold-water fish (rich sources of EPA and DHA) and enjoy a very low incidence of degenerative disease, led researchers to study the workings of these two highly unsaturated fatty acids in the body. It was determined that EPA and DHA help lower the melting point of the saturated fats, thus keeping them from attaching themselves to arterial walls.

The world's leading authority on the omega-3 fatty acids present in marine oils is acknowledged

71

to be the brilliant Danish professor, J. Dyerberg, M.D., Ph.D. Dr. Dyerberg heads the Department of Clinical Chemistry at the Aalborg Hospital (Aalborg, Denmark) and is responsible for a number of landmark papers on the effects of the polyunsaturated fatty acids, particularly in the treatment and prevention of atherosclerosis.

Dr. Dyerberg has an explanation for the failure of most nutritional authorities to recommend the daily intake of marine oils until recently. He says, "Fish oils were originally not mentioned in most dietary guidelines to lower serum cholesterol and prevent atherosclerosis. One reason for this might be that the populations most concerned with preventing atherosclerotic diseases do not readily accept and enjoy eating seafood. Another reason is that the long-chain polyunsaturated fats have low melting points and are easily oxidized. These qualities create problems in the manufacture of margarine and shortening. Reports published in the 1950s and 1960s indicating that fish oil may lower blood cholesterol even more than vegetable oil, had no major impact on early dietary recommendations. The first real breakthrough concerning dietary fats occurred with the report of the clinical effects on coronary atherosclerosis of a diet rich in seafood."

In conjunction with H.O. Bang, it was Dr. Dyerberg who initiated the dietary studies of the

Greenland Eskimos in the late 1970s. This report was published in 1981 in *Acta Scandinavia* Vol. 210: 245-248. Building on earlier research, the scientists uncovered the reason for the very low incidence of cardiovascular disease in Eskimo society. Although the population ate a very high fat diet (known to promote heart disease) of whale, seal, and walrus meat, they universally consumed a lot of cold-water fish as well.

After expanding his study to include Greenlanders, Dr. Dyer explains, "Statistics from Greenland show a low mortality rate from ischemic heart disease (atherosclerosis) with no sex difference. From 45 to 64 years of age, 25 out of 277 male deaths (9 percent) and 13 out of 178 female deaths (7 percent), or 38 out of 455 deaths (8.4 percent) both sexes were recorded in a 5-year period within a population of approximately 50,000. In the community of 2000 inhabitants, 10 years of medical records did not include a single death from ischemic heart disease."

Within the last few decades, cardiovascular disease has risen steadily in Japan. As the Japanese people have embraced western dietary preferences in place of their-traditionally high consumption of fish, the rate of death from cardiovascular disease has kept pace. As they have dropped fish from the menu and patronize McDonald's instead, the Japanese no longer enjoy their previous immunity from heart disease. Western disease patterns are now apparent in the population of Japan.

Most of us would not find a daily diet of fish palatable. It would be difficult for the typical American to choke down the amount of fish that gives the Eskimos their seeming immunity to heart disease. However, a Dutch scientist, D. Kromhout recognized the problems such a diet would pose to the western world and had a study already in progress to determine exactly what quantity of fish a person would have to eat to enjoy its protective effect. The results of Kromhout's study were published in the *New England Journal of Medicine* in 1985. Here's what he found:

In order to calculate the relationship between the measured intake of fish and coronary mortality, Kromhout selectively chose a group of 852 middle-aged men whose dietary habits could be determined for the 20-year period of the study. He assigned risk factors according to the amount of fish normally consumed. Men who disliked fish and never ate it, were found to have a risk factor of 1.0. Those men eating from 1 to 14 grams of fish had a risk factor of 0.64; those consuming 15 to 29 grams had a risk factor of 0.56; and those eating 30 to 144 grams had a risk factor of 0.36. After reviewing Kromhout's data, Dr. Dyerberg noted, "The interesting observation made by Kromhout is the inverse relationship between a relatively low level of fish intake and coronary heart disease. This finding makes nutritional advice based on the seafood hypothesis much easier to give and accept, compared to that based on data from Greenland and Japan which describe fish intakes that are unrealistically high for many people."

HEART HEALTH & MUCH MORE—Both EPA and DHA are present in the most important and active organs and tissues of the body, including the brain cells, the nervous system, and the sex glands. The omega-3 fatty acids play a very important part in regulating the chemical balance of the body and assist in normalizing the coagulation factor of the blood. In impressive double-blind clinical studies, fish oil has been shown to possess remarkable arterial-cleansing ability. It has reduced cholesterol and triglyceride levels, significantly lowered dangerously high blood pressure, eased the pain of rheumatoid arthritis, worked against migraines, and has even shown protective effects against cancer.

Cardiologists and doctors all over the world are now prescribing fish oils as a proven therapeutic measure for those with dangerously high cholesterol and triglyceride readings. In clinical tests, omega-3 fish oils were shown to almost miraculously lower harmful blood fats, while increasing beneficial blood fats that protect against heart disease.

In the *New England Journal of Medicine,* Dr. Michael Davidson of St. Luke's Medical Center reported on a study of patients taking fish oil capsules which showed spectacular results. Over-all cholesterol levels dropped 24% and triglyceride levels fell 48%. Dr. Davidson pointed out that simply taking fish oil capsules cut the risk of suffering a fatal heart attack by 50% for those patients.

Important Health Tips

1) While many adults need to be on a restricted cholesterol diet, children do not. Children from infants to pre-teens could actually be harmed from such curtailments in their eating patterns. They need all the nutrients their bodies can receive for healthy bone growth, cell formation, and the accelerated body growth which are an integral part of childhood.

2) *Unrefined, cold-pressed flaxseed (linseed) oil* is a wonderful supplement for those trying to lower their cholesterol. In addition to the benefits already listed in this chapter, there is increasing evidence that flaxseed oil may enhance the body's immune system, which would help to make your system more resistant to a host of illnesses and chronic conditions.

But, keep in mind that you should also be using other equally *healthy vegetable oils when you cook and in salads.* Don't throw those health benefits away by using polyunsaturated fats. Some of the best oils for these purposes are olive, safflower, sunflower, and other oils made from whole seeds.

Do not use flaxseed oil for cooking, because the heating process will destroy the enzymes and the good health qualities found in this "golden" oil.

ESSENTIAL FATTY ACIDS CONTENT
OF COMMON VEGETABLE OILS

Source	Fat Content Total%	Essential Fatty Acids Linolenic	Linoleic	Both Essentials Total %
Flaxseed	35	58	14	72
Soybean	18	9	50	59
Pumpkin	47	15	42	57
Walnut	60	5	51	56
Rapeseed*	30	7	30	37
Safflower	59	0	75	
Sunflower	47	0	65	
Grape	Trace	0	71	
Corn	4	0	59	
Wheat Germ	10	0	54	
Sesame	49	0	54	
Rice Bran	10	0	35	
Cotton**	Trace	0	50	
Peanut***	47	0	29	
Almond	54	0	17	
Macadamia	71	0	10	
Cashew	41	0	6	
Olive	20	0	8	
Coconut	35	0	3	
Palm Kernel	35	0	3	

*	Rapeseed (canola) contains toxic *erucic acid*
**	Cottonseed contains common toxins
*** Peanuts (damp) harbor a toxic fungus

Hemp (not listed because it is illegal in the U.S.)provides both essential fatty acids.

Nature's Cholesterol Blocker

Diet modification is the best way to lower cholesterol. However, it isn't always easy to change years of poor eating habits. Even those of us with the best of intentions sometimes have trouble staying away from some types of foods.

Now there is great news. Two new, all-natural supplements, recently developed, may help lower your cholesterol, while you are in the process of changing your eating habits.

They are *LoCholest*™ and *Ventrux Acido*, which represent major breakthroughs in health care technology. When taken together, you may be able to block a significant portion of the cholesterol in your diet from being absorbed in the body and restore the functioning of your intestinal flora and bowel movement.

The recent discovery of a group of natural substances in common plants has led to a new generation of powerful, natural cholesterol-control compounds that are completely safe and remarkably effective. Modern technology has concentrated these substances into an easy-to-take tablet that blocks cholesterol absorption during a meal. One tablet of *LoCholest*™ and *Ventrux Acido* taken with your meals may prevent the accumulation of excessive cholesterol.

Of course, some cholesterol, as we noted earlier, is essential to the proper functioning of the body. According to the experts, a person needs between 250 and 300 mgs of cholesterol daily. This is far less than the 500 to 2,000 mg the average person consumes daily.

Ventrux Acido helps maintain the health of your intestinal tract through the maintenance of normal, beneficial intestinal flora. These help to "unclog" your digestive system, which allows the stomach to function even more efficiently by digesting the foods more completely. This results in more and better quality nutrients for your body's use.

This product has been regorously tested and found safe and effective. It's all natural formula can be taken by everyone, regardless of age, without fear of any adverse side effects.

Similarly, *LoCholest*™ has met the high standards required and also has been found to be a natural, effective way to lower cholesterol. In medical double blind studies, doctors tested both men and women who had normal to high readings. Double blind tests involve one group receiving the product being tested, in this case *LoCholest*™, while the other group is administered a placebo, a pill which has no beneficial qualities.

Each group, given the natural plant substances, found in *LoCholest*™, experienced a 20 to 64 percent decreased absorption rate, according to test results.

LoCholest™ has been compared to a group of trained detectives which move through the intestinal tract seeking out cholesterol molecules. Once found, they become attached to *LoCholest*™ and are carried out of the system— long before they can begin to harm the body in any way.

This process in no way impairs the absorption of essential nutrients. Many cholesterol rich foods, in fact, are the best sources of protein, complex carbohydrates, as well as vitamins and minerals.

In fact, the combination of *LoCholest*™ and *Ventrux Acido,* may actually ensure a higher absorption rate of the nutrients essential to the body's daily functioning, while blocking the absorption of excess choleserol.

Both products are available through *Biowell,* whose address is listed in the end of the book.

Natural Ways to Lower Cholesterol

Method	Suggested Dose
Alfalfa	Daily salad with alfalfa sprouts included or 4 tablets with each meal of the day (12 tablets daily)
Calcium Pectate	2 medium carrots daily or 1 cup chopped cabbage daily 1 cup chopped onion daily
Cardiosan™	A proven European formula to strengthen the heart One capsule daily
Vitamin E	800 International Units Daily
Flaxseed Oil (unrefined only)	1 to 2 tablespoons daily
Garlic *Garlimed*™	1 clove daily or 3 tablets daily
Healthy Bones	A powerful calcium supplement, 2-6 capsules daily
LoCholest™	3 tablets daily, lowers cholesterol almost immediately
Magnesium	400 mg daily
Oat Bran	1-1/2 to 3 oz. daily
Pectin	10 grams daily (1 medium-sized apple contains two grams)
Dr. Rinse Formula	1 to 2 tablespoons daily

"Good" Cholesterol's Beneficial Role In Fighting Disease by Clearing The Arteries of Deadly Plaque.

"What's your number?" is the latest educational campaign to make people more aware of the importance of their cholesterol level.

It may not be too long before people will be asking, instead, "What's your ratio?" as the importance of "good" cholesterol emerges.

Good and bad cholesterol are what they are called. Simple terms, but very descriptive. Low Density Lipoproteins or LDLs are the "bad" variety. These are the type that register when you have your cholesterol level tested.

And up until very recently, these were the only kind that really mattered to the medical community.

But, enter the good guy. High Density Lipoproteins (HDLs) are the beneficial type of cholesterol and act much like a "bouncer" in a night club—they escort the bad guys out. (For a detailed account of how this happens see the illustration on page 86).

And, medical researchers are now saying that the more HDL a person has, the more protection he has from atherosclerosis, also called hardening of the arteries, or plaque build-up.

In fact, Dr. Meir J. Stampfer of Harvard Medical School, told a conference of the Amercian Heart Association recently, "If I was going to know just one number, it would be HDL."

Dr. William Castelli, of the Framingham, Mass. study, which has followed a community's patterns of heart disease for some 20 years, thinks the best indication of risk of heart attack is a ratio of the total cholesterol to the HDL.

For example, if you had a cholesterol reading of 180, and an HDL level of 60, your ratio would be 3.

The more HDL to your overall level, the better your protection, in other words, the lower the ratio, the better.

A ratio of 4.5 or higher could put you at a fairly high risk of developing heart disease, Dr. Castelli noted.

With this system, vegetarians have among the lowest ratio at 2.5, with marathon runners, next with 3.4.

The average female victim of heart disease, Dr. Castelli continued, has a cholesterol ratio of between 4.6 to 6.4, while male heart patients average between 5.4 to 6.1.

A higher ratio indicates a strong possibility that plaque has already formed on the arteries' walls and atherosclerosis may already have taken hold of your blood vessels. Atherosclerosis, a relatively slow process, carries with it dangerous health implications. Complete blockage of the arteries present the very real potential of a heart attack.

Medical researchers are investigating the possible health benefits derived from raising HDL in the blood. Would an increased level remove the plaque already built up on the arteries? Researchers believe this just might be so.

A recent study conducted by Dr. David Blankenhorn, director of atherosclerosis research at the University of Southern California, demonstrated that in some cases, at least, obstructed arterial walls benefited by exposure to greater numbers of HDLs.

Researchers are also looking into the possibility of synthesizing this good cholesterol. If this could be done, it may be an effective treatment for heart patients and a viable alternative to the oftentimes harsh drugs they must take.

But that option is still a few years away. Until then, the best health advice anyone can give a person is to be aware of his cholesterol count and take steps to maintain a healthy reading, or to reach that level if yours is too high. This can be accomplished by following certain dietary guidelines.

In the following chapters, we'll provide you with some secrets of nature, which will help you in the struggle to overcome high cholesterol and may prevent or reverse atherosclerosis and other related health problems and heart diseases.

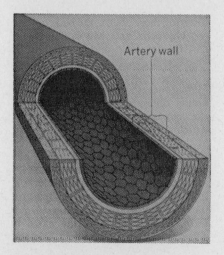

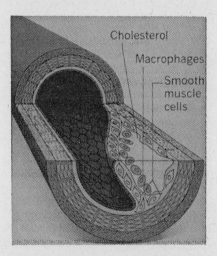

Healthly Artery
Undamaged inner walls allow for free flow of blood.

Diseased Artery
Heavy plaque buildup narrows the opening and restricts flow of blood.

"Good" Cholesterol's Beneficial Role In Fighting Disease by Clearing The Arteries of Deadly Plaque.

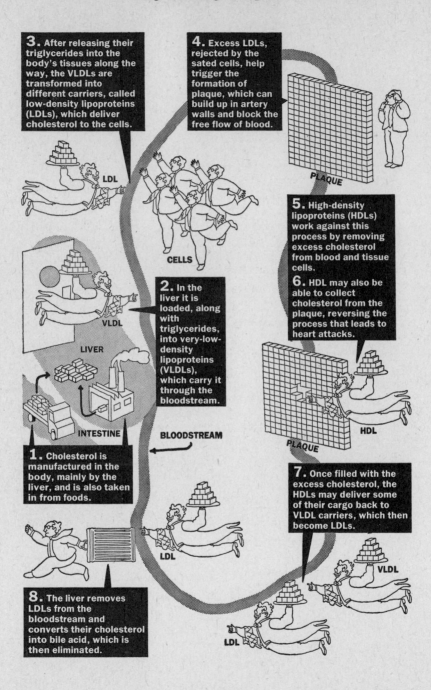

3. After releasing their triglycerides into the body's tissues along the way, the VLDLs are transformed into different carriers, called low-density lipoproteins (LDLs), which deliver cholesterol to the cells.

4. Excess LDLs, rejected by the sated cells, help trigger the formation of plaque, which can build up in artery walls and block the free flow of blood.

5. High-density lipoproteins (HDLs) work against this process by removing excess cholesterol from blood and tissue cells.

6. HDL may also be able to collect cholesterol from the plaque, reversing the process that leads to heart attacks.

2. In the liver it is loaded, along with triglycerides, into very-low-density lipoproteins (VLDLs), which carry it through the bloodstream.

1. Cholesterol is manufactured in the body, mainly by the liver, and is also taken in from foods.

7. Once filled with the excess cholesterol, the HDLs may deliver some of their cargo back to VLDL carriers, which then become LDLs.

8. The liver removes LDLs from the bloodstream and converts their cholesterol into bile acid, which is then eliminated.

LDL

VLDL

LIVER

INTESTINE

BLOODSTREAM

CELLS

PLAQUE

PLAQUE

HDL

LDL

VLDL

LDL

Chapter 3

The Effects of Cholesterol

The majority of us think of an artery as a pipe which allows for the passage of blood, similar to the pipes in our bathroom that supply water to our sink and bathtub. But arteries are much more than pipes. They are *living, self-repairing organs* that work as biochemical "factories" for enzyme systems.

When a person reaches his late 40s and early 50s, enzyme production gradually declines, which is a contributing factor to atherosclerosis, according to heart specialists. The enzyme system acts as a natural barrier against hardening of the arteries.

As their production declines, the formation of atherosclerotic plaque—lumpy, thickening of the interior of the arterial wall—increases. The cells' lining grows rough. These developments narrow the size of the passageway and may, indeed, provide sites for the formation of blood clots which can diminish the flow of blood even more.

The plaque deteriorates into ulcers containing

calcium deposits which attract blood clots. These ever-increasing impediments to freely flowing blood frequently block the vessels completely.

A blocked artery may damage several parts of the body. If the vessels that supply blood to the heart are involved, a heart attack results; if the cerebral arteries are blocked, the person will suffer a stroke. Gradual blockage of the arteries, doctors explain, may cause senility—a slow loss of memory and deterioration of the mind. Arteries providing blood to the kidney can also be affected by athero-sclerosis. A blockage in this area causes Bright's Disease which produces swelling and eventual kidney failure.

Signals of Arterial Degeneration

Atherosclerosis is not a localized condition, it's effects are not limited to one part of the body. Rather, the entire human body is affected by hardening of the arteries. The sad aspect is that atherosclerosis seldom announces itself until it is too late to do much about it.

But, there are some signals that should alert one to the possibilities that his arteries may be clogging. It's a fact that every person who suffered a fatal heart attack had *some symptoms or sign of* warning of the approaching event. It may have been a tightness in the chest, a pain in the left jaw or an ache in the left shoulder. Most commonly, one of these symptoms will *occur when this person is under stress*. We will discuss a few of the symptoms which should alert one to problems.

Intermittent Claudication

Intermittent claudication, cramping in one or both legs during physical activity, is a symptom of artery problems. This is not to be confused with the occasional leg cramps one gets while resting or sleeping. Rather, it affects one as he begins to walk, indicating an inadequate arterial blood supply to the leg muscles. Intermittent claudication seldom occurs as a result of standing, sitting, or reclining.

Intermittent claudication, in rare instances, can occur in the ankle, feet, toes, forearm or wrist. Claudication has been known to occur in a single finger as well. Experiencing claudication in the feet feels as if one is walking on gravel or cobblestones.

As time passes, cramping—no matter what area of the body is affected—becomes more painful until physical activity is severely restricted.

Claudication is usually accompanied by other warning signs of impaired circulation, such as varicose veins, swelling or numbness of an extremity or localized pallor. Moreover, a lessening or even an absence of pulses in the arteries above the feet may be noticed.

Pulses Lessened

A lessening of the pulses in the feet is indeed a signal of possible arterial damage. There are two pulse locations in the foot. The first is on the instep approximately four inches below the big toe. The second is on the inner side of the foot at the point the Achilles tendon slides past the ankle bone. If you cannot find a pulse in either location, try to locate one behind the knee or along the thigh in the groin. When feeling for a pulse, it's best to use the tips of the three middle fingers.

While you're locating your pulses, also examine the skin of the lower limbs for abnormal distribution of temperature. A normal skin temperature indicates an adequate arterial flow. Warm skin does not always mean something is wrong, however. *Cold skin is a sign of an inadequate arterial flow.* Cold feet will be pale or even blue or purple. The darker the color of the feet, the more serious the problem.

Each of your legs should be the same temperature. Feel the area over the knees and the front of the thigh as well as its inner portion.

Transient Ischemic Attacks

A transient ischemic attack is a recurrent episode of neurologic impairment, which can last from several seconds to several hours. It is a warning sign of an impending stroke.

Symptoms of such an attack include double vision, slurring of speech, temporary loss of vision called *fleeting blindness,* staggering or an uncoordinated walk, weakness or numbness, dizziness and falling due to weakness in the legs.

The flow of blood is temporarily decreased because of *microemboli*—small blood clots—have congregated in a localized area usually at a rough spot of the artery. They may fleck off occasionally into the internal neck artery or some other blood vessel. The symptoms one displays depends upon the area of the circulatory system in which the clots are lodged.

The middle cerebral artery is composed of main branches which go to the brain hemispheres. A blockage causing decreased circulation to the middle cerebral hemisphere, therefore, may cause weakness in the arm or the loss of control in the fingers. If the dominant cerebral hemisphere experiences decreased oxygen flow, the situation may manifest in a lessened ability to express oneself. Slurred speech results when the non-dominant hemisphere lacks sufficient blood flow.

Skin Color and Hardening of the Arteries

The color of one's skin is indicative of arterial flow. Thomas Lewis, M.D., has outlined how to judge changes in skin color as they relate to hardening of the arteries.

Warm, Pale Skin. Indicates a rapid flow and an abundant supply of fully-oxygenated blood. The skin is pale because it is well nourished and the minute vessel tone is high.

Warm, Deeply-Colored Skin. The skin is in a state of inflammation, having been irritated by heat or other causes. It may also mean the skin has been arterially dilated from drugs or by nervous channels in the body.

Cold, Pale-Bluish Skin. The flow of blood in this instance is very slow or even absent. If the skin is tinted violet or blanched, the circulation is absent and has been arrested for several minutes.

Cold, Deeply-Colored Bluish Skin. The circulation is very slow and, in fact, blood flow has been failing for sometime. The skin may also show a process of low grade inflammation.

Cold, Deeply Colored Red Skin. Very cool skin, such as this, is usually about 50 degrees Fahrenheit, and does not want to part with its oxygen. This serious coolness damages the minute vessels by holding them in prolonged dilation.

CHAPTER 4

The World-Famous Dr. Rinse Formula

To Prevent Or Reverse Hardening Of The Arteries And Heart Problems.

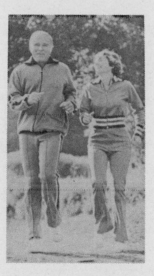

This amazing formula, developed by Dr. Rinse for his personal use after an incapacitating heart attack, has enabled tens of thousands of individuals around the world to overcome heart disease. Empirical evidence in the form of testimonials from grateful users shows the Dr. Rinse Formula not only aids in the fight against cardiovascular and circulatory problems by cleaning out arteries clogged with cholesterol, but can reduce high blood pressure and even ease the pain of arthritis.

I became personally acquainted with Jacobus Rinse one crisp Sunday afternoon in the middle of his vast acreage in a remote corner of Vermont. My wife and I motored up from our home to have dinner at his invitation. We drove leisurely, thoroughly enjoying our passage through the rolling hills of Ohio, ablaze with the changing colors of autumn, up through the majestic mountains of Pennsylvania crowned with snow-caps and wreathed with hazy clouds of snow.

Following the good doctor's excellent directions, we finally reached the Rinse holdings and turned into the lane. As we drove down what has to get the longest "driveway" I ever traveled, we heard the sound of a chain-saw echoing across the river. As we continued driving down the lane, the sound got louder and we were busy looking around trying to spot the operator through the trees when the saw noise stopped.

Suddenly, coming across the river toward the road, there appeared Dr. Jacobus Rinse. I stopped the car and walked eagerly to greet him. I found it hard to believe this alert, vigorous man, coming toward me with the welcoming smile, was 88 years old. His stride was that of a much younger man and the chain-saw in his hand testified to his afternoon's occupation. "Just clearing out some dead wood," he explained. "I was cutting it into lengths to fit the fireplace and stacking it into cords.

After a very pleasant and convivial meal, I expressed my surprise and complimented him on his excellent physical condition. Even though I had read his published works and many of the articles written about him, I still was amazed to think he had transformed himself from a semi-invalid who, according to his medical prognosis, should have been dead long ago, into the dynamo seated before me.

He chuckled a little and told us a bit about his schedule. On many occasions, he said, he climbs into his old Volkswagen and makes the four-hour trip down to New York City in his capacity as chemical consultant. Upon arriving in the city, he may give a lecture, attend a luncheon or participate in a meeting. Without staying overnight or pausing to rest, he then climbs into the VW and makes the four-hour return trip. Dr. Rinse regularly works until 2:00 in the morning and boasts, in his words, "a heart as sound as a child's."

Although many people are unaware of it, the Dr. Rinse Formula he developed, and which has helped so many overcome their health problems, brings him no income. This remarkable man has no remuneration whatsoever. It is strictly an altruistic effort. Dr. Jacobus Rinse is a benefactor of mankind and, as a healer, knows no peer.

When asked if he had any secrets, he smiled in reply. "No secrets. Proper nutrition, suitable exercise and my formula, that's all." Dr. Rinse says emphatically, "Anyone can have the same results."

In The Beginning

Thirty-seven years ago, after suffering his first heart attack at the age of 51, Dr. Jacobus Rinse was told he had ten years to live—provided he restricted all physical activity and took his prescribed medications daily. Remembering the sharp pain and agonizing vice-like constriction of the chest he experienced during his heart seizure, which followed an unusually active weekend clearing the land where his new house was to stand, Dr. Rinse resolved to follow the orders of his cardiologist to the letter. With his very life at stake, he had too much to lose to take any chances whatsoever. His life as a virtual invalid began.

Born and educated in Holland and holding a doctorate in physical chemistry, Dr. Rinse couldn't understand what factors had combined to create his heart condition. As a textbook case, he didn't fit. By medical standards, he should not have been a candidate for early heart problems. He knew that individuals at risk usually have a family history of heart disease, that many smoke, and that most are overweight and eat a diet high in cholesterol. Dr. Rinse was the first member of his family to experience a heart attack, He had never smoked, and watched his diet, virtually eliminating foods targeted as high in cholesterol, such as eggs, butter, most dairy products and fatty meats. Other contributing factors to heart disease are thought to include physical strain to the breaking point and emotional stress or excitement continuing over a period of time. He examined his life and found these criteria did not apply to him either.

Yet, in spite of his healthy lifestyle, his angina attack was the very real result of an atherosclerotic condition characterized by cholesterol-clogged arteries. Popping nitroglycerin pellets, sometimes as often as every fifteen or thirty minutes, to open up the constricted arteries, which caused his heart to spasm painfully, was not to his liking. Dr. Rinse explains, "I was not satisfied to make use of these small pellets for the rest of my life—even if it was only to be 10 years."

As a practicing research chemist, Dr. Rinse was

determined to change his body chemistry and reverse his prognosis. He investigated natural foods thought to protect against cholesterol buildup and began eating raw foods rich in fat-liquifying enzymes. From 1951 when he suffered his first heart failure until 1957, he lived on raw fruits, raw vegetables, raw herring, raw meat, raw eggs and yogurt. He began taking 1000 mg of Vitamin C (ascorbic acid) daily and a multivitamin tablet. Being aware of the research of Evan Shute, M.D. and Wilfrid E. Shute, M.D. of Ontario, Canada, who successfully treated many heart patients with Vitman E, he determined to follow their recommendations and began taking 200 mg of Vitamin E after meals.

During this period, Dr Rinse relates that the one single supplement he felt helped him best tolerate increased physical activity was *garlic*. Talking of the rigid regimen he set for himself and followed without deviation for six long years, Dr. Rinse now says,"by avoiding overly strenuous exercise, I managed to live a more or less normal life."

However, his satisfactions were few and in 1957, he experienced another excruciating attack, lasting an agonizing hour this time.

He suffered almost constant spasms of angina pain, in spite of his medication. His heart-rate rose an alarming 50 beats and he was slow to recover after the slightest amount of exercise. It was beginning to appear the medical experts were right after all.

With six years of his precious projected ten gone, Dr. Rinse refused to be conquered and began his serious research all over again. There had to be a key.

Certain scientific tests conducted on laboratory animals with chemically-induced high cholesterol levels came to his attention. This research indicated the substance *lecithin*, derived from soybeans, could actually dissolve cholesterol. In addition, *safflower oil* was shown to contain precisely the polyunsaturated fatty acids needed to reduce cholesterol to a liquid state. Could it be possible that a combination of lecithin and safflower oil would conquer atherosclerosis in humans and clear clogged arteries? Dr. Rinse decided to find out, using himself as a guinea pig.

Along with his other supplements, he began to take one tablespoon each of lecithin and safflower oil daily. Incredible as it may sound, in only a few days, he began to feel the difference as his body responded.

Dr. Rinse reported, "My angina pains ceased. My galloping pulse rate decreased slightly, but noticeable. Excellent results began to appear within a few days." After three months of continued use,

99

his angina symptoms totally disappeared, even after exercise. The chemist in him attributed his improvement to the lecithin and safflower oil.

One short year later, his physical activity now encompassing even heavy outside work, his condition appeared completely cured. Dr. Rinse explained, "I am convinced the food supplement I developed is both a preventive and cure for atherosclerosis. I have had no recurrence of angina or other diseases. It seems the atherosclerotic plaques which had been narrowing my arteries to cause heart failure have been reversed."

Judging from his extraordinary health at 88 years of age, Dr. Jacobus Rinse was completely correct. He has personally conquered one of the major killers of our time.

The Dr. Rinse Formula
A Personal Account

Recently, my mother-in-law, 74, frail, with a weak heart, suffering from atherosclerosis and angina pain, crippled and all but incapacitated by arthritis and osteoporosis, took it into her sweet stubborn head to leave her native Bavaria and come to the United States to visit us. My wife was frantic with worry over her condition and certain the trip would end with our having to put her in a hospital. She prayed only that it wouldn't happen in route, with Nan-Nan being rushed on an emergency basis to a hospital in some distant city.

We tried every which way to change Nan-Nan's mind, including several very long-distance phone calls, but it didn't matter to her that we had a trip scheduled to see her the coming autumn and offered to escort her back with us; it didn't matter to her that her health really wasn't up to such a long trip and she refused to confront the possibility of a fall which could result in broken bones already weakened by her osteoporosis.

Osteoporosis is a very common condition in the elderly, especially those living alone. It is caused by a disturbance of the body's metabolism resulting from a deficiency of certain nutrients and minerals (primarily calcium), usually present in an adequate diet. But, like many senior citizens, Nan-Nan's family had scattered. With no one to cook for but herself, we were sure she had lost interest in food and and no longer bothered to serve herself a balanced meal. Without the elements they need to keep strong, bone mass and density decrease, the bone becomes honeycombed with too much air space and osteoporosis progresses rapidly. Such bones are brittle, fragile and break very easily.

Nan-Nan had already undergone two separate operations for joint replacement when her brittle bones had snapped and would not heal. She was in

101

constant pain from angina and the osteoporosis, and favored her right side when she walked, creating a back problem as well.

Nan-Nan's angina attacks required strong medication to bring the pain to bearable levels. The coronary insufficiency she labored under was caused by an advanced case of atherosclerosis, commonly called "hardening of the arteries," often making her short of breath as her heart labored to send oxygenated blood where it was needed. With the blood flow to her heart slowed by constricted and every-narrowing blood vessels, she was a prime candidate for a heart attack, stroke or other degenerative condition—all of which come from atherosclerosis.

Add to that the swollen joints and nodules of the arthritis that cruelly curled her hands and sent pains shooting through her body and you can well understand why we were worried about Nan-Nan making such a long trip alone.

Always indomitable, Nan-Nan let us know she was determined to come alone now—and that's exactly what she did. The relief was evident on my wife's face when we met the plane and she could finally put her arms around the tiny hobbling figure and support her to the car. Her face was gray with the fatigue of the long flight, but we got her home and I tucked her up warm and cozy while my wife went to fetch a cup of herb tea and honey for all of us.

Leaving them to chat a little, I took my tea downstairs to my favorite chair and began to think seriously about Nan-Nan's medical problems. Certainly it was going to be easy to make sure she had an adequate diet while she was with us, but she refused to leave her home and live with any of her children. What would happen to her health when she went back home? What single one thing could we do for her that was simple and easy enough for her to continue when she returned to Bavaria? What could we do in the four short months of her visit that would make enough difference in the way she felt so that she would want to continue it herself? Suddenly it came to me! Nan-Nan would join us in taking the *Dr. Rinse Formula breakfast-mash* every day.

Two years before, when I was entering my 50s, I found I was slowing down and I didn't like it. I had always followed what are generally considered good health practices and enjoyed robust good health for the whole of my life, but I suddenly found myself puffing going up the stairs and continually fell asleep after dinner. Although there wasn't anything I could really put my finger on, except shortness-of-breath and lack of energy, I took myself to the doctor. He joked I was "just getting old," but put me through a complete battery of tests. He found my cholesterol levels were elevated above the normal range and talked to me about "hardening of the arteries" and what medical problems atherosclerosis could create.

In 1983, I had presented "The Dr. Rinse Formula" to my readers. I was personally very impressed with the good doctor and his natural, almost-miraculous cures of atherosclerosis, high (and low) blood pressure, arthritis, bursitis, phlebitis, angina and more. I recalled such a flood of letters from grateful individuals testifying joyously to their renewed well-being and health after taking Dr. Rinse's Formula.It created a happy problem— that of selecting just a few to excerpt for publication!

From that time on, my wife and I began taking Dr. Rinse's breakfast-mash religiously. My cholesterol reading fell dramatically and I have the boundless energy of a child again. My wife glows and the twinges of early arthritis she was experiencing have vanished. Apparently we had caught ourselves in time, but what about Nan-Nan? Could Dr. Rinse's Formula help such a diversity of medical problems all concentrated in one frail old body.

YES! The very next morning, with a little urging from my wife, Nan-Nan downed her portion of Dr. Rinse's Formula and dutifully took the alfalfa tablets I laid out for her. Although her problems were of very long-standing, I am absolutely delighted to report that within just two weeks, changes in her condition were noticeable. Her breathing was no longer labored and she seemed to be getting around more comfortable. Within two short months, she was able to help around the house—and enjoyed it thoroughly. By the time she left to return home after four months with us, she was freely moving her fingers without pain for the first time in eight years, thanks to the Rinse Formula and the alfalfa tablets.

It is impossible to fully describe the dramatic changes Dr. Rinse's Formula worked for Nan-Nan. We brought home a fragile, stooped lady suffering from a seemingly impossible conglomeration of ills and sent home a relatively spry, happy, oldster looking forward to life again! Her last letter says she is doing marvelously and confirms she will never be without her breakfast-mash. I, for one, am not surprised! Chalk up another victory for Dr. Rinse.

Dr. Rinse's Formula
Praised By Many

Here's a small sampling from our Files:

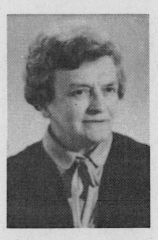

Mrs. Elizabeth Bouse
Housewife
Trenton, New Jersey

Mrs. Bouse, 74 years old, tells us she had been afflicted with swelling of her hands and knuckles and was unable to do any housework for many years. Atherosclerosis and arthritis affected both her knees so severely, she was barely able to move around. Even daily chores were beyond her. When a friend told her about it, Mrs. Bouse started taking the Dr. Rinse Formula and three alfalfa tablets three times daily. Her condition began to improve in just two weeks. After two more weeks, her fingers became more flexible and she lost the stiffness in her knees. She was very happy to be able to move around more freely, and now rejoices in being able to do her own housework again! After three months on the Dr. Rinse diet, all her symptoms disappeared and she was able to do her daily chores without pain for the first time in many, many years. Mrs. Bouse's doctor was amazed at her improvement and he's now recommending this diet to his patients with similar conditions.

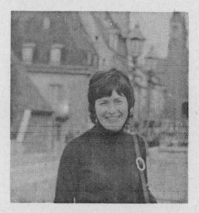

Mrs. Trudy Wein
Billings, Montana

When I turned 40, my doctor put me on medication for various disorders, such as atherosclerosis, arthritis and hypoglycemia (low blood sugar). My blood pressure was always very low and I suffered from cold hands and feet for many years. My fingers and toes felt numb most of the time, except when the arthritic pain caused my fingers to swell and hurt. I took a strong medication which helped my condition somewhat, but at the same time, I became very dizzy, couldn't sleep, had migraine headaches and a sinus condition. A friend of mine read your book and told me about the incredible results she had experienced just by taking the Dr. Rinse breakfast mash. She convinced me. After only a month, I could see the first signs of improvement myself, I'm 45 now and have been using the Dr. Rinse formula for six months. All my symptoms have completely vanished! I can't believe the difference. I can run up the stairs without puffing, my hands and feet are always warm, and my doctor discontinued my medication. Even my cholesterol level is normal. I'm very thankful for this improvement. My doctor now gives me a

107

clean and perfect bill of health. I'm full of energy and everyone thinks I look about ten years younger!

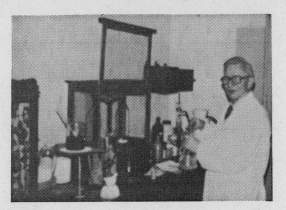

Professor
Dr. Armin
Hoelscher, Ph.D.
Chemist and
Retired
St. Petersburg
Florida

This 84-year old professional man had severe angina, heart problems, poor blood circulation, very low blood pressure and a high cholesterol level, as well as other serious cardio-vascular-related ailments. Dr. Hoelscher was unable to walk more than few hundred yards without stopping frequently to catch his breath. He suffered an artery blockage in his lower right extremities, causing him severe pain. He was forced to drag his right leg as he walked. He was on Lanicor for many years to stabilize his failing heart. After using the Dr. Rinse Formula for just four weeks, he wrote us to say he could feel his symptoms slowly diminishing. After three months on the Dr. Rinse mash, the Professor was able to breathe more freely, could walk up steps without problems and even resumed his morning walks for the first time in many years. After two more months on the mash, Dr. Hoelscher wrote again to tell us of his joy at being able to walk up to two miles daily and do some vigorous exercise and heavy outdoor work. We were especially pleased to hear from this scientist. As a pharmacist and chemist, he was skeptical at first, but is now convinced. What all his other medications were unable to do, the all-natural Dr. Rinse Formula accomplished by providing him all the essentials he needed to stabilize his health.

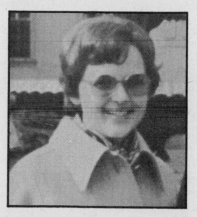

Crystal Fannes
Executive Secretary
Palm Beach, California

At my age of 51, I had always been basically in very good health. But, without any warning, I developed a severe pain in my back caused by blockage of one of my arteries. I also had a very high cholesterol level. While riding in the car with my husband, I suddenly fainted and he rushed me to the hospital. They diagnosed me as having lack of oxygen to the brain, caused by poor circulation. Even my breathing was irregular. My doctor warned me I was a prime candidate for a heart attack if I didn't change my diet. But the medication he gave me seemed to make me feel even worse. I was always tired and had no energy. The world around me was gloomy. After I read about the Dr. Rinse Formula, I mixed it up myself at home and it took only two weeks for me to show improvement. After I had taken the Formula for about four months, I was able to drive again without fear. My family is certainly glad I regained my old happy disposition. I'm not taking my prescribed medication anymore. I don't need it since I've been using Dr. Rinse's mash every day at breakfast. I can't find words strong enough to tell you how thankful I am for your book. I'm full of energy now. My doctor was very surprised to see how fast I recovered my excellent health on the Dr. Rinse Formula.

A.M.H.
Chemist
Borger, Texas

I am 70 years old and hold the equivalent to a major in biology form the University of Missouri. I was the Chief Chemist for Phillip Petroleum during my professional career and am now retired. After reading about Dr. Rinse, I started taking his formula in 1973 with about 2 teaspoons of soy lecithin granules and 1-1/2 teaspoons of safflower oil each morning for breakfast. The mixture was supposed to keep cholesterol in solution so it would not form a slime in the blood vessel which could break loose and plug an artery. At this writing, I have cut back to a rounded teaspoon of lecithin and 1 teaspoon of oil.

After about two years on the Formula, my doctor asked me what I was doing. He said my blood tests were like an 18 year old's! After my regular physical exam two years later, he again expressed amazement at my blood tests. After two more years on the breakfast-mash, I took a physical in Temple, Texas and they said the same!

This formula is so good, it should be publicized to help humanity!

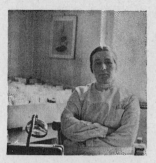

Elna Groth, N.D.
Naturopathic Physician
Austria

This naturally-oriented health-care professional writes:
I'm using strictly homeopathic medicine to take care of my
patients' health problems. But sometimes homeopathy doesn't
give lasting results and I'm always searching for better
treatment for my patients' ailments. While on vacation a few
years ago in the U.S., I learned of the Dr. Rinse formula and
have since used it on may hundreds of my patients suffering
health conditions that don't normally respond well to any
medication. I have seen the most wonderful results with this
mixture of vitamins in such cases as heart disease, angina
and other coronary problems. Many of my patients afflicted
with arthritis, gout, varicose veins, high cholesterol and even
eye disorders, such as glaucoma, have responded favorable.
I, myself, have been using Dr. Rinse's mash for almost two
years. I must say I feel more energetic and positively reju-
venated! My blood pressure, always a problem, is now nor-
malized.

Based on the incredible results I have seen in my patients
and the studies on nutrition I have been doing, I feel this
formula can overcome the hardships of disease and save
many lives. The Dr. Rinse Formula may well be considered a
universal health formula for many ailments. I can highly
praise it from my own experience. Every person of middle-age
should consider the Dr. Rinse mash daily. I believe it may
ward off a lot of ailments that might otherwise occur. Dr.
Rinse has developed a good, wholesome, natural preventive
medicine of the finest kind.

111

THE DR. RINSE FORMULA

The Proportions Given Below Will Make a 14-Day Supply

7 Tablespoons Lecithin granules
6 Tablespoons raw Wheat Germ
6 tablespoons debittered Brewer's Yeast
    (powder or flakes)
6 Tablespoons Sunflower Seeds
6 teaspoons Bonemeal from a reliable source
    (powder or tablets)
6 Vitamin C tablets of 0.5 grams each
6 Vitamin E tablets (200 International Units total)

To These Ingredients, I Also Add:

6 Tablespoons Bran Flakes
    (for better bowel movement)

6 Teaspoons Kelp powder
    (or 6-12 Kelp tablets)

Zinc 150 mg

All seeds or tablets should first be crushed in a blender.

Blend these ingredients well in a big bowl, stirring until the mixture is uniform. For improved health, take 1 to 2 Tablespoons of the Formula on a daily basis. To insure freshness and complete potency of all ingredients, I recommend you store your Dr. Rinse Formula in a closely covered jar in the refrigerator.

This formula comes pre-packed in 14 oz cans (two week supply) available from Biowell. (See last Page of Book)

Closing Comments

You may also add a good dollop (about 1 table-spoon) of raw, unheated, unfiltered honey. You may use molasses, if you prefer. The honey or molasses should be added at the time you swallow the mixture. A good morning regimen also includes a multi-vitamin/mineral tablet and three to five natural alfalfa tablets. When selecting your alfalfa tablets, be sure to secure then from a good reliable source. *Biowell* is a good source for healthy vitamins.

As "heart-health" maintenance, you might take 1 tablespoon daily of the Dr. Rinse Formula to create the catalytic effect for your heart. In case of heart disease, arthritis, rheumatism, osteoporosis, gout or combination conditions, such as Nan-Nan suffered, be sure to take five of six alfalfa tablets three times daily. Alfalfa helps wash out toxins that have built up over the years and adds minerals needed by the body to repair damaged cell tissue.

Many people take the Dr. Rinse breakfast mash as a tasty addition to their morning cereal. As a change of pace, use it to top yogurt or blend it into a high-protein shake. If you don't mind a somewhat "lumpy" drink, you may also stir it into any juice, such as grape, orange, pineapple or my favorite, cranberry.

113

Besides being a good natural "energizer," honey is one of nature's most powerful germ killers. Harmful bacteria cannot survive in raw honey. Primitive man made this discovery and used honey both as a sweet treat and as a salve to heal wounds. And, did you know that honey used as a sweetener doesn't result in the production of heavy body fat, as does refined sugar? Honey is delicious and digestible, as well as being nutritious. In fact, many nutrition experts consider honey a supplier of power for the heart muscle itself! If you prefer Dr. Rinse's Formula sweetened, you may add honey with a heavy hand and a clear conscience!

Once you start taking the Formula, don't be impatient! Although it is true some individuals seem to experience almost immediate relief, *plan on allowing three months before* the results become perceptible to you — and be pleasantly surprised if it happens sooner! After six months on the Formula, its therapeutic value will be quite apparent and you will surely be on your way to better all-around health.

Even if you're not suffering from atherosclerosis, arthritis, hypertension (high blood pressure) or are not at risk of cardiovascular disease, I promise the Dr. Rinse Formula will improve the quality of your health and give you so much rip-roaring energy, you'll feel like a frisky kid again.

The World Responds

Letters began flooding Dr. Rinse's mailbox the moment the world discovered the wonderful benefits of his formula. The gratitude and praise has not stopped. People from just about every industrialized nation have been helped through this amazing mixture. Literally thousands of lives have been saved and many more restored to health, through the dogged determination of Dr. Rinse.

Mr. B.L. of Des Moines, Iowa:

I had severe high blood pressure for 10 years. After only six months on the formula, my blood pressure now averages 125 over 80. Not bad for a 65-year old. I feel 15 years younger. I work hard and play hard and once again really enjoy life."

Mrs. Faith J. Trenton, New Jersey:

"The doctor told me I had poor circulation. On top of that I suffered from arthritis. If that wasn't enough, I constantly felt tired and even my eyesight was growing worse. If this was old age creeping up on me, I wanted no part of it. Within two weeks, all that began to change, thanks to the doctor's formula. I noticed an increase in my stamina, a lessening of my arthritic pain, even an improvement in my vision. Today my life is far more active than my children's.

Mr. Vince G., Atlanta, Ga.:

"My medication for my heart problem gave me so much pain I couldn't take it. Someone suggested the Dr. Rinse formula. After nine months, the pain stopped. I'm 67 years old, but I don't feel a day over 40. Thank you, Dr. Rinse.

Mrs. B.L., Baarn, Netherlands:

"My atherosclerosis was so bad, I had to stop working. But that was six months ago. Today I'm back at work— even working overtime—because of what the Dr. Rinse Formula did for my body. It was a Godsend."

Mr. Ron C., San Antonia, Texas:

"I took the directions for the Dr. Rinse formula to my own physician. He wholeheartedly endorsed my plan of action. He said he had been using it for years to help control his own blood pressure.

Mrs. D. Penn, Red Oak, Iowa

"The results I have obtained with your formula were startling. In just 16 days my blood pressure dropped noticeably. My angina pains are all but gone. After two months, I could exercise with no pain."

Mr. Merle W., New Haven, Conn.

"Fantastic. That's all I can say about the Dr. Rinse Formula. Before I took it, I felt like an old man. I had high blood pressure, was short of breath, frequently became dizzy and had extremely poor circulation in my arms and legs. That's all history now. All my complaints vanished. In fact, people marvel these days about my energy and vitality. It's not so bad being 68 years old."

Following are examples of recipes using the Dr. Rinse Formula:

MELON (or other fruit) SHAKE

½ cup chunks of cantaloupe & honeydew
¼ cup plain yogurt or lowfat milk
1-2 teaspoon(s) fructose
1 oz. Dr. Rinse Formula

Mix in blender, first at low then high speed until completely liquified.

BANANA MASH

1 large ripe banana
1 packet fructose or 1 tsp. honey
1 oz. Dr. Rinse formula
3 tbsps. lowfat milk

Combine ingredients & mash with fork until consistency of pudding (smaller portion: medium banana & ½ oz. of Dr. Rinse Formula).

117

MOCHA NUT COOLER

6 oz. lowfat milk
½ tsp. instant coffee
½ tsp. chocolate extract
¼ tsp. almond (or other
    nut) extract
1 tsp. honey or fructose
1 oz. Dr. Rinse Formula

Blend at high speed for
one minute.

HOT CHOCOLATE
MUG-A-LUG

¾ cup hot chocolate drink
½ tsp. vanilla extract
1 oz. Dr. Rinse Formula

Prepare hot chocolate
drink. While hot, pour into
blender with other ingre-
dients. Blend at high
speed for one minute.

DR. RINSE PANCAKES

¾ cup whole-wheat
    pastry flour
4 tbsps. Dr. Rinse Formula
½ tsp. salt
½ tbsp. brown sugar
½ tsp. baking powder
1 egg (optional)
1 tbsp. safflower oil (for
    pan)
½ cup skim milk

Measure whole-wheat
pastry flour, Dr. Rinse
Formula, salt and brown
sugar. Beat an egg and
add milk to the egg. Add
egg mixture to the dry
mixture. If a thinner pancake

is desired, omit the egg or
add more milk.
Brown pancakes in the
safflower oil. Add more oil
if necessary. Serves two
(two 4-inch pancakes each).

APPLE BUTTER SPREAD

6 tbsps. apple butter
¼ tsp. cinnamon
1 oz. Dr. Rinse Formula

Place all ingredients in bowl
and mix thoroughly with a
fork. Use as spread or eat as
you would a pudding.

BRAN MUFFINS a la
DR. RINSE

10 tbsps. Dr. Rinse Formula
1 cup whole-wheat flour
1½ cups coarse bran
1 tsp. baking soda
½ tsp. cinnamon
½ tsp. grated orange rind
¼ tsp. cloves
few gratings of nutmeg
1 egg
1/3 cup blackstrap molasses
½ cup raisins soaked in
    ¾ cup hot water

Combine all dry ingredients.
Beat the egg with the
liquid from the raisins and
add the molasses to this
mixture. Combine the two
mixtures. Add the raisins.
Bake in buttered muffin tins
for 20 minutes at 350°.

Yield: one dozen muffins.

Chapter 5

A New Break-through Formula From Denmark

" I think living is a beautiful experience."
—Pohl Nielson after
experiencing rejuvenation with Longo Vital®

Pohl Nielson had spent 12 years of his life laying flat on his back in his bed. In that time his bones had grown together, making him stiff. He could not bend and could barely manage to raise himself from his bed to make one meal daily. He suffered pain constantly.

That was before *Longo Vital*®, the very special all natural remedy from Denmark. Within a month Pohl discovered he had the ability to stand for several hours without pain. While he is still unable to bend his body, the constant pain subsided dramatically and he manages to garden—his first love—and to perform odd jobs around the house.

"Now I can climb up. It is slow but I manage—

and when I reach the top step, I can decide if I want to paint the house or make a speech," Pohl said. One could not fault him if he decided to make a speech. He said it "would be a speech of praise. Because I got up by myself and am standing there in the fresh air with a view of the fields, our own little house and the garden where I know every flower..this is everything I have ever dreamed..far more than I have dared hope for the past many years."

Most of us don't have the severe health problems Pohl does. We can move about without too much trouble and our bodies bend when we need them to. But, if *Longo Vital*® can transform a man who had been laying—almost dead—for a dozen years into an active, vital human being, think of the wondrous changes it can bring to your life.

Long Vital® is an all-natural nutritional supplement developed by one of Denmark's—and the world's—leading medical doctors, Flemming Norgaard, M.D., D.D.S. He was the first person in Denmark to earn two doctorate degrees, one as a medical doctor and the other in the field of ondotology—the study of the health and structure of the teeth. Moreover, his honors are unparalled in his native Denmark—with a host of honorary degrees and other distinctions.

Longo Vital® naturally activates the body's own

120

often hidden abilities to work at peak performance and to heal itself.

Gunnar Askerheim discovered that. "Fifteen years ago" he said, "I developed rheumatic pains. It grew progressively worse over a seven-year period. My joints became swollen and I had considerable difficulty moving about. Cortisone was of no help, but Dr. Norgaard's *Longo Vital*® special formula did help. The pain I had lived with for so long vanished quickly—almost magically—and now I feel strong and well again."

Longo Vital® increases the energy level and provides vitality for the elderly. But it is also of tremendous benefit to the young and middle-aged person. One of its best qualities in this fast-paced world is to give one a feeling of calm and control in times of stress. In fact, this specially developed natural supplement has already provided thousands of people all across the European continent a higher interest and enthusiasm in their jobs. They enjoy their time away from work even more since they began taking this supplement and have used this marvelous opportunity to actually live life—not just go through the motions.

This synergistic blend of all natural ingredients works by renewing cells and activating the vital cell functions. Cells need proper nutrition for their health, including a balance of trace elements which are easily absorbed by the human body

In fact, a well-balanced diet is an absolute necessity for robust health, yet few of us seem to receive one. After all, poor eating habits can lead to many illnesses, including heart disease. *Longo Vital®* can help. Let's face it, our diet most of the time just doesn't measure up. And while doctors may scold their patients, up until now little could be done about it.

Longo Vital®, though, can help you overcome the results of poor eating habits—habits which medical authorities now say contribute to premature aging and the onset of many chronic diseases mankind is now plagued with.

If you're like many of us, you're probably listening to your doctor and making an honest effort to improve. But is isn't easy. The addition of *Longo Vital®* into your diet, can help ensure your health—even on those days when you fall back into old poor eating patterns.

This natural supplement will aid your body in feeling healthier, help your cells grow and work better so that you have more energy. And once you start feeling better, you'll find that your body will literally begin to crave fresh fruits and vegetables and other nutritious foods. *Longo Vital®* gives your body a chance to grow healthy. A chance is usually all it needs.

122

Mrs. Ulla Lindon, 43, gave her body the opportunity to choose health. "I developed bald patches
all over my head," she related. "My hair fell off in
large chunks. Since I was not taking any medication, I realized that my diet must be deficient. I tried
Longo Vital®. My hair came back very quickly and
even my nails began to grow again."

Harriet Longquist had been bothered for several
years with recurring colds. The 60-year old tried
the natural tablets. She no longer battles colds.
And her nails grow healthy, long and beautiful
now. But Mrs. Longquist was most surprised by
her improved vision.

Immune System Strengthened

Longo Vital® is able to promote these changes
in people because of its unique ability to
invigorate the body's natural immune system.
This natural Danish supplement hastens the
healing process of damaged cells, which then
delays the death of the organism. This makes it
easier for the body to fight off diseases and
infections—even the ever-elusive viral
infection.

In fact, scientific studies have confirmed that
more than 80 percent of those people who now use
Longo Vital® regularly have a significant improvement in the ability of the immune systems to fight

diseases.

Viruses have the ability to alter their form according to Dr, Norgaard and, thus, it is practically impossible to create a vaccination for them. "A vaccine for one type of virus will not be effective for a slightly different type," he explained. But, with *Longo Vital®*, the body's immune system is strengthened to help naturally eliminate the virus.

"When I feel as if I'm coming down with a cold or the flu," the doctor said, I take six of the tablets in the morning instead of usually three—and I don't get sick."

One of the most stubborn of all viruses is the one responsible for Herpes Simplex I and II. Doctors struggle to control the outbreaks of herpes—keeping them to a minimum. There is no known cure for the disease. But regular use of *Longo Vital®* can indeed help control the outbreaks. "Even the most severe and resistant cases of herpes," the doctor said, have been alleviated with regular use of the *Longo Vital®* supplement.

People who have suffered with treatments for six and eight years with no real results found relief with the all-natural formula. These cases, according to Dr. Norgaard, "had been given up as hopeless" by doctors and the best of clinics around the world.

Laura K. experienced a very persistent case of herpes. She suffered with visible eruptions up to four times a month. Her case was so bad, even her lymph nodes swelled. Laura had given up hope— after all she had visited all the best doctors.

Then a friend suggested *Longo Vital®*. She tried it but didn't hold out much hope. How could three tablets a day help her when all the best physicians of Europe were at a loss?

In about a month, her herpes had improved tremendously. She has used the formula and has not experienced a recurrence of eruptions. Dr. Norgaard states: "This doesn't mean we claim to cure these cases. It's well known that viruses lie hidden in the nervous system. If one's resistance is lowered for any reason, the lesions could recur."

However, if one follows the recommended dosage of three tablets per day, the herpes indeed may be controlled. It's important, though, that one take the supplement even if he is feeling great and has not experienced an outbreak in awhile. If one discontinues using *Longo Vital®*, the herpes will reappear.

Improves Cardiovascular System

Longo Vital® may help one prevent the occurrence of cardiovascular and heart disease. Many people have reported their continued use of this natural remedy actually lowered their blood pressure. The Danish supplement acts as a mild vasodilator—which means that it helps enlarge the vessels so more blood can flow through. For people who are afflicted with hardening of the arteries, whose vessels are clogged with cholesterol, this could, indeed, mean a world of difference in their health. People have even said that their chest pains, caused by coronary sclerosis have subsided dramatically.

"I was amazed to discover that after only using *Longo Vital®* for a week, my pulse rate lowered quite a bit," said Terry Hirgelt, a professional writer. "I had changed nothing else in my life—my diet was the same and I didn't increase my exercise habits. Yet my pulse was slower. This excited me and I am now taking my exercise more seriously, as well as my eating habits along with my daily *Longo Vital®* tablets. The way I see it, the combination of these can surely work miracles on my body."

And don't think that just because you haven't reached your 50s and 60s yet that you don't have to worry about heart disease. It's a slow gradual process. Heart and cardiovascular conditions do not just suddenly appear—they are the culmination of a lifelong deteriorating process. In fact, medical experts say that the first degenerative

126

signs of aging in the vascular system—and other areas of the body as well—begin to show between the ages of 30 and 35 years. One is still young at this age. But if you begin supplementing your diet with *Longo Vital®* when you are in your 30s, then the odds are high that you'll be one of the lucky people who can avoid heart disease. At the very least, using *Longo Vital®* at the relatively young age of 33 will give you more energy.

Aging Process Slowed

An added bonus is starting off with this natural supplement early in life is the slowing of the aging process. *Longo Vital®* has counteracted the complaints which usually accompany old age—drying of the skin, brittle nails, and dry, lifeless hair to name just a few of the problems.

Karen Lundholm was 76 years old. She was depressed and continually felt tired. In fact, it was not unusual for her to stay in bed until noon. Karen felt little joy in living—and had little purpose to live. Some days she would get out of bed just to make a meal, then head back for the bedroom and get under the covers again. It was almost as if she were hiding from life.

She noticed, moreover, that she was losing her hair. "I had always been so pleased with my hair.

It had always been so thick and strong. So it was very upsetting when it suddenly started to fall out in large chunks."

It was Karen's hairdresser, concerned about the amount of hair Karen was losing, who suggested *Longo Vital®.*

"I must say what happened was nothing short of a miracle. The first thing I noticed was that *I became almost terribly bright.*" She no longer stayed in bed till noon. In fact, she began rising at 6 a.m. again, as she used to do.

Her hair began to grow again! This pleased her immensely. "It started to grow like mad," Karen recalled. Even the eczema, which Karen had experienced for several years was gone after taking *Longo Vital®.*

"I have suddenly become very pleased with myself in my declining years," she exclaimed.

Gertrude Jacobson recognizes the changes Karen underwent. She read about *Longo Vital®* and gave the all natural formula a try. There was nothing specifically wrong with her. But she said that her disposition is much more pleasant now. She acknowledges everyone may not receive the same dramatic results so fast, but is amazed that it has transformed every elderly person she knows who has taken it regularly.

Urinary Infection Relieved

Mrs. Sigrid Fallenius suffered from depression. "I tried all sorts of medicine," she said, "but received no results." Then she discovered *Longo Vital®*. She became cheerful again. "I was alert and extroverted again," she said with a song in her voice, "not tired and apathetic as I had been previously."

Mrs. Gidget Setterberg, too, was amazed at the efficiency of the specially formulated *Longo Vital®* "I was always bothered with urinary tract infections," she said. "I was also plagued with arthritis. Naturally, I was worried about my future. With these conditions, it didn't look too bright. Every prescription, the doctor wrote was stronger than the previous one. I was worried about what this medicine was doing to my system."

A friend told her about Dr. Norgaard's special synergistic formula. "I figured I had little to lose. It was safe to take with my medicine so I thought I would buy two bottles. If I noticed no improvement after using two bottles," Mrs. Setterberg remarked, "I could stop taking these supplements. At least it gave me hope."

Hope is not the only thing *Long Vital®* gave Mrs. Setterberg. "I got well," she stated simply. No more urinary tract infections. No more arthritis pain.

"But I am staying on this supplement to be sure I stay free of any problems," she explained.

Herbert Christenden felt as if he constantly had a cold and a sore throat. It was irritating, but he knew it was more serious than that. Herbert felt his body was trying to tell him that it was in need of help. His body's natural defenses, he realized, were somehow lacking. But he didn't know what to do to improve the situation.

"My sister, who's a nurse, advised me to take *Longo Vital®* for my infections. I was skeptical at first. After all, it wasn't medicine, but just a natural supplement. How could it help me?" Herbert wondered.

But it did! "Now I am hardly ever ill! And my hair and nails grow tremendously," he said.

You may wonder why everyone has experienced hair and nail growth. This growth is indicative of the cell rejuvenating process occurring throughout your body. Just as *Longo Vital®* restores health to your hair and nails, it is restoring health to every part of your body. "You can be sure the same effect (healthy growth) is occurring in the many other tissues and organs of your body" explains Dr. Norgaard.

Luis Nilsson has no doubt about the marvelous powers of *Longo Vital®.* "My wounds heal so much faster now," he said. Luis is a carpenter, so getting cut and scraped is an occupational hazard.

Incontinence Cured

Mary C. was a normal, happy young lady in her mid-20s—until she inexplicably developed a severe case of incontinence. It is an embarrassing problem and her specific case began to get worse. Soon she dared not even go out of the house.

This medical problem, which no doctor seemed able to cure, crushed her emotionally. If she feared leaving her house, she knew that her hopes of ever having a loving family of her own were gone forever.

Mary turned from her happy outgoing self into a depressed recluse - until a friend persuaded her to try Dr. Norgaard's *Longo Vital®* tablets. She was extremely skeptical. "How could these silly tablets, help me," she asked her friend, "When all the doctors in Europe have failed?"

But her friend was persistent. Mary finally agreed to try the natural tablets if only to prove her friend wrong. However, it was Mary who was the one that was surprised. The formula worked. In a very short time, Mary noticed a slight improvement. With each day, the changes for the better became greater.

131

Soon this young lady was able to confidently appear in public and enjoyed social functions once again. She even started dating.

Mary discovered that happy endings really do happen. Today she is married and has a loving young son. Her life dramatically improved because of *Longo Vital®*. Of course she is still taking the natural supplement today, as is her husband. It's a safe bet that their child will have two very energetic parents as he grows up.

The Dr. Norgaard Story

Dr. Flemming Norgaard is not your average doctor. He is a very extraordinary human being dedicated to helping others. Just look at the number of honors his peers have bestowed upon him.

Professor Flemming Norgaard, M.D., D.D.S.
F.R.C.R., F.R.S.M., F.B.I.R., F.A.C.R., M.D.R.G.,
F.M.S.R., M.N.S.R., M.D.S.D.R. (Honary)
Honorary Secretary/Treasurer International Society
Radiology Emeritus

In fact, a scientific society dedicated to the advancement of odontolgy bears his name. His research in this area laid the foundation for the current treatment of patients who have problems with their temples.

132

"Without my work, today's treatment would be impossible," Dr. Norgaard noted quietly. His discoveries in this field were not met with critical acclaim overnight, however. It took 13 long years before the majority of the medical community recognized and valued his achievements.

His latest original research deals with arthritis. He has devised a method of diagnosing arthritis up to 10 years before its actual onset. With this information, many people may be saved the agony of suffering with this often times unbearable condition.

In addition to this intensive research, Dr. Norgaard also devoted himself to his patients. He spent over 25 years as a senior doctor at one of the leading hospitals in Copenhagen, Denmark. He left only to start his own private clinic to continue to help people overcome illness and diseases. So he knows the pain and surffering patients endure at times. It was this concern that prompted him and two other physicians, in fact, to found an international league of radiologists where knowledge can be shared to benefit all. Dr. Norgaard was instrumental in arranging for many conferences and congresses that brought together some of the most talented and brightest people in this field.

To look at this tall, energetic man, now 81 years old, its hard to believe he was ever ill—or even

133

tired—a day in his life. But he was. He spent too many years complaining of fatigue brought on by a doctor's erratic schedule and the heavy pressures of dealing with people's lives.

"I had finished my work at the hospital," Dr. Norgaard explained, "and had started a major private practice which soon became too much for me to handle. I was exhausted."

"I was so tired and ill that I could not cope with anything at all. I consulted my colleagues. They gave me a thorough examination and believed my problem was simply I was growing old and literally dying from over exertion."

He refused to accept that diagnosis, however, and turned his insightful research abilities toward discovering something which would relieve his fatigue. It did not take this remarkable man very long. *Longo Vital*® is the culmination of years of research and rigorous scientific testing. The synergistic blend of natural ingredients transformed Dr. Norgaard from a tired old man to an enthusiastic, exciting gentleman.

To give you an idea of this man's natural reserve of energy, Dr. Norgaard's latest visit to the United States several months ago was a fast paced two weeks. He gave lectures, led seminars to many groups on the East Coast and in the Midwest. Additionally, he spent several days in Washington,

D.C. with a colleague discussing their extensive correspondence on medical and research matters. On most days he was on the go before 6 a.m. and never stopped before 7 p.m.

Even his wife has benefited from *Longo Vital®*. Mrs. Norgaard, in her husband's words "became younger and even more beautiful" after only a month of using the natural tablets. The changes in her, though, went much deeper than appearances. Both the doctor and his wife were surprised—but delighted—to discover a significant improvement in her chronic abdominal disorders. She had used just about every type of medicine available for her problems, but none seemed to effectively rid her body of pain. She had taken so much medication, in fact, that Mrs. Norgaard wondered at one point if her troubles actually stemmed from the disorder or from the flood of drugs to which she had been subjected.

With *Longo Vital®* , she needed the medication no longer. The symptoms had disappeared and the elated woman thought her husband a magician.

Not A Medicine

It must be emphasized here that *Longo Vital®* is not a medicine. It is not a drug nor any type of medication. Rather it is a natural, nutritional supplement, which when taken as directed, provides this body with the needed substances for robust health. Perhaps if we could travel back in time to the days before processed and refined foods, we would not need *Longo Vital®* . But we can't. In our hectic times, these foods are a convenience which the majority of us have grown to depend upon. It's sad but very true. *Longo Vital®*, however, can quickly and efficiently restore the missing ingredients for good health. And it does it naturally.

Not every supplement works for every person. And it just may be that these tablets may not provide you with the energized feeling that most people experience. But the odds are so great that you will find the relief and the love of living that *Longo Vital®* should be your first choice. For a mere 60 cents a day, you can discover if the *Longo Vital®* multi-potent special formula works for you. It's an inexpensive and low risk method.

Most people feel a change almost immediately. Some feel a difference after a couple of days and for others the noticed improvement takes a week or so. If after six to eight weeks of faithful *Longo Vital®* use, you feel no improvement, either in a specific condition or in your general well being then you can discontinue using them. After this length of time, you can safely assume that your problems are of an origin different than what *Longo Vital®* can do.

Amazingly Effective Longo Vital®

Longo Vital® has already helped thousands of people across the European continent. This synergistic all-natural new formula offers a great feeling of energy and vitality few people have ever experienced. The most wonderful aspect is that it is achieved through a gentle, natural approach whose effects are long lasting when this scientifically developed formula is taken as directed.

Dr. Norgaard's Longo Vital formulation can act as a wonderful natural aid for many disorders of the body, as well. Listed below are just some case histories of health conditions which have been alleviated, according to the Danish doctor's experience and findings:

- Relieves stressful conditions
- Lifts Depression
- Rebuilds ailing bodies and tissues
- Strengthens nails, hair and skin
- Lessens severity of menstrual pain
- Alleviates problems associated with menopause
- Normalizes functioning of prostate gland
- Overcomes incontinence
- Relieves certain cases of psoriasis
- Helps with arthritic-like conditions

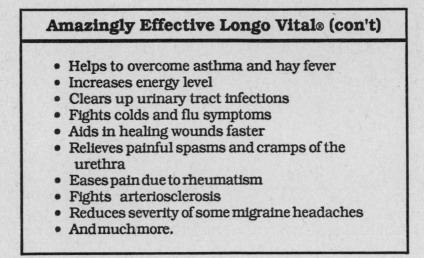

Amazingly Effective Longo Vital® (con't)

- Helps to overcome asthma and hay fever
- Increases energy level
- Clears up urinary tract infections
- Fights colds and flu symptoms
- Aids in healing wounds faster
- Relieves painful spasms and cramps of the urethra
- Eases pain due to rheumatism
- Fights arteriosclerosis
- Reduces severity of some migraine headaches
- And much more.

Recommended Dosage of Longo Vital®

First Week: 3 tablets with Breakfast
3 tablets with Lunch

If you *do not feel* and improvement in your general well-being continue this dosage for the second week.

If you *do feel* positive signs that your ailment is responding to your new strengthened immune system then follow this lowered maintenance dosage:

***From the
Second Week on:*** 3 tablets with Breakfast

138

If after six to eight weeks you still feel no response from the all-natural *Longo Vital®* formulation, stop using it. It very well may be that the origin of your condition lies elsewhere and medical attention may be required.

The moment you feel as if you're coming down with a cold or the flu, then increase the dosage of these tablets to between six and eight daily for a few days. By that time, the signs of an impending cold should have disappeared and you may return to your three daily tablets.

The same procedure can be followed for those times when you feel especially filled with tension. If you have a stressful event coming up, your dosage may be increased.

There is no danger in doing this for several days in a row. ***Do not, however, continue this practice beyond a week or 10 days.***

There are no side effects due to the natural ingredients of this supplement. *Also, it is safe for diabetics.* When you take an extra dose because you are stressed or ill, you may, however, find you will actually need less sleep than usual. *Dr. Norgaard cautions against taking the pills in the late afternoon, because some people may experience trouble falling asleep that night.*

*Longo Vital®*can be taken with any type of medication—either prescription or over the counter.

Chapter 6

A Very Special Exercise Program To Help Maintain A Healthy Cholesterol Level And Strengthen The Heart

When combined with the suggestions in the previous chapters, exercise can be a valuable tool in lowering your cholesterol level and in building a stronger and healthier heart.

Among the many benefits of participating in a physical activity include boosting of the immune system through an increasing lymph flow, improving the respiratory functions, slowing the aging process and increasing the flow or richly-oxygenated blood to every single cell in your body.

The American Heart Association, the American Cancer Society and many other widely respected health organizations, all recognize the

141

need for a regular exercise program in reducing your chances of acquiring many diseases, including heart disease and atherosclerosis.

Experts explain that a person's fitness level peaks in his early 20s and normally declines as he ages. But, those who exercise regularly can keep that fitness level higher for many more years than inactive people.

In fact, data on those individuals who lived to be more than 100 years old, show that they had one thing in common. They all performed hard physical labor on a daily basis. Studies show that many of these people had "silent" heart disease, but the physical demands they placed on their bodies protected them from developing fatal heart attacks.

Rebounding As An Efficient Exercise

There are many different exercise programs which would benefit your heart. You may choose from among walking, jogging, bicycling to name just a few. All will help lower your cholesterol as well as increase the health of your heart.

We would like to introduce you to another activity which may not be familiar to you, but is an excellent choice. If you are serious about your health, you will want to investigate rebounding.

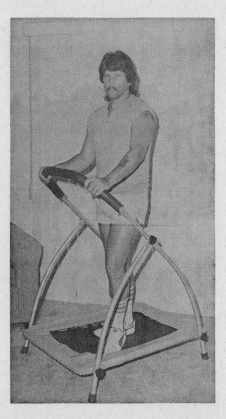

It's easy to rebound! An excellent way to increase your circulation, this activity may improve your overall health and keep your organs functioning properly. Performing this easy exercise regularly, may also help contribute to normalizing your cholesterol level and strengthening your heart, thus adding extra protection against heart disease and atherosclerosis, and other related life threatening diseases.

143

Rebounding is an exercise performed on a personal-sized trampoline. You may jog in place on the rebounder, jump or perform a variety of simple routines. In evaluating this form of activity, NASA found it to be 68 percent more efficient than jogging.

Why Rebounding Is So Effective

When you jump regularly on the Rebounder for as little as 10 minutes daily, every cell in your body changes and improves. The basic physiological changes go by a variety of names: cardiovascular enhancement, increased aerobic capacity, improved stamina or endurance. But they all mean the same thing: A healthier you.

Most forms of exercise concentrate only on certain body parts, requiring the participant to incorporate more than one form of workout into his program in order to fully exercise the entire body. *Only rebounding exercises the entire body all at once* by subjecting each cell to increased G-Force (Gravity).

One of the effects suffered by astronauts, directly caused by the weightlessness of space travel was a measurable loss of bone mass. Their bone cells responded to the absence of gravity by reducing bone density. These cells "knew" almost instantaneously that they no longer needed the

144

strength required to oppose gravity.

Another effect of space travel, documented by Swiss scientists, was a marked inhibition of the immune system. After examining the white blood cells (lymphocytes and leukocytes) of both American and Soviet space travelers these researchers subjected the weakened cells to added G-Force.

They confirmed that these important immune system cells responded to increased gravity by becoming even stronger and more active than under normal earth gravity.

Rebounding is the only activity which subjects the body to this phenomenon, thereby stimulating the extremely important immune system defense of the body which is vital to our resisting diseases and ailments of all kinds.

In rebounding, the added effects of acceleration and deceleration come into play, as well. On the downward bounce, the added G-Force painlessly stresses every single cell in the body. Each cell responds by strengthening itself almost immediately.

As each cell responds to this increase activity, possible only in this exercise, it becomes stronger. The whole body benefits dramatically. Rebounding exercises the entire body—all at once—not just a single part. Every cell gets a real workout. And that's very important.

145

Test The Difference

If clinical findings and scientific facts aren't enough to convince you that rebounding is the most universally effective form of exercise ever devised by man, try this test yourself.

Sit on the floor with your legs extended straight out before you. Place your hands at rest on your lap. Have another person place his hand on your chest and push you backwards. Without using your hands for support, resist with all your might. You'll find that no matter how strong you think you are, you can't hold yourself up.

Now hop on to the Rebounder and vigorously jog in place for only three minutes. Then return to your original position on the floor, legs stretched out straight in front of you. Ask the same person to push you backwards again. Resist as you did before.

Because every single cell in your body has instantaneously responded to the increased physical demands of the increased G-Force caused by rebounding, you will find that you are dynamically strengthened and can very easily remain upright.

The Facts of Life

Fact I   Most rebound units are not built well enough to support a consistent exercise program longer than 30 days.

Fact II   NASA evaluated rebounding and found it to be 68 percent more efficient than jogging, generally considered to be one of the best aerobic exercises.

Fact III   Rebounding helps more than just your heart. This unique activity also aids in improving body balance, coordination, rhythm, timing, and dexterity, as well as strengthening muscles.

Fact IV   Rebounding, the most efficient and effective form of exercise ever devised by man, can be performed in the privacy of your home or office in any time of weather. And it's the perfect activity for all ages, from adolescent on up.

At The Forefront of Technology

The exercise programs outlined in this chapter will provide you with all you will need to increase the flow of blood to your heart and every organ in your body. Moreover, the program may very well help to control your cholesterol level.

The regimen provides the lowest impact stress available in exercise today. And it is designed, if carried out regularly, to increase your aerobic capacity, which increases your heart strength and function of all your cells in the Body.

It is the first rebounder to incorporate hand rails (for safety and easy use), plus an engineering design rectangular shape with air-shock-absorbing mat to assure even tension and bounce. These safety features make this rebounder an effective device for an at-home total exercise regimen.

In the past, I did not regard rebounders with enthusiasm, because I felt their construction was poor, even dangerous. The cheap, poorly-constructed versions can still be found at mass merchandising outlets throughout the country. These bind, tear, and break. Often, accidents occur with some danger to the user. Well, all that has ended with the Rebounder. It is constructed from aircraft aluminum; the pad is made of polypropylene memory yarn that doesn't stretch and sag (a common complaint with other Bounders), and it has steel reinforced, resilient rubber components—I mean, it's safe to use! This piece of equipment is designed to last.

Why should you exercise on the Rebounder? Let me tell you.

A Low Impact Highly Effective Exerciser

Rebounding exercise traces its origins to the trampoline, which was invented in 1936. During World War II, trampolining became a popular form of exercise that was used to develop balance, coordination, rhythm, and timing. Athletes soon discovered the trampoline. To this day, pole vaulters, gymnasts, runners, wrestlers, soccer players, volleyballers, skiers and others use the trampoline to develop their athletic skills.

The value of the trampoline as an exerciser for developing the body was not overlooked either. During the 1950's, trampolines were used in physical education classes in many junior high and high schools. However, without certified supervisors and because of daredevil users, the trampoline made an early exit from the schools. Although trampoline centers sprang up around the country in the early 1960's, with trampolining promoted as a form of recreational exercise, a lack of real information and qualified supervision made the apparatus nothing more than a high-flying bouncer.

It was not until the late 1970's that the first home-sized rebounder appeared in its early form. Incorrectly called a mini-trampoline, the rebounder has stiffer springs than a true trampoline and isn't used to achieve a high spring. The purpose of a rebounder is to absorb the shock of your

149

body weight as you move up and down in low bounces. The 1980's have witnessed the technological development of the rebounder into a more useable and effective training machine.

We studied the engineering aspects of this equipment with the aim of making it a durable, indestructible, safe exercise device. We also studied the use of the rebounder and have developed this exerciser to accommodate a wide range of users and a multitude of exercises. I have developed a program of exercises, presented a little further on. But, first I want to tell you why you should exercise on the Bounder.

It takes the stress out of running, jogging and walking—any movement where your body weight exerts a force on your joints, tendons, ligaments, and muscles. Rebounding helps you fight and overcome gravity, but allows you to exercise your cardiovascular system and your muscles. And, thanks to modern technology, you can reach your target heart rate and monitor your energy expenditure with a simple inexpensive watch.

I consider Rebounding an ideal warmup exercise, because you don't feel the soreness that one often experiences when beginning a run. Rebounding quickly gets your blood moving, giving you a muscle pump, and it's a nice feeling! Once you get going each exercise builds on the previous one, giving you a sensational feeling that you have "worked" your muscles. There's an enthusiasm you develop with this form of activity that doesn't occur with other exercisers.

Early on, this can cause you to get winded by being too aggressive especially if your muscles can last longer than your aerobic capacity. However, your endurance level quickly improves and overtraining doesn't occur. The Bounder "tells" you when you have had enough.

Rebounding can be used to exercise specific muscles, too, especially the hard-to-develop leg muscles—calves, ankles, thighs, and feet. I mention feet because there are many foot injuries today among athletes and active people that are caused by weakened bones and joints. So, it's not surprising that rebounding can be used to help rehabilitate injuries. The activity provides low-impact exercise so you can exert a minimum amount of force and stress, something you can't do when running or bicycling. And, perhaps the added gravity force provided by rebounding increases the output of endorphins. You'll really feel better after you have worked out for even as little as 10 minutes.

The actual exercise uses of Rebounding are broad-based. You can lose weight, trading fat for lean body weight. Energy expenditure can be as high as 200 calories per ten minutes in your target heart rate exertion! And, because you can build

151

muscle with this simple exercise, you can actually gain lean body weight by rebounding. It is an excellent adjunct to the exercise regimen of athletes, also. You can achieve a muscle toning you can't derive from other forms of exercise.

But its primary use is an exercise program for the active person. Many people don't want to go to a gym or club, and really can spend only ten minutes on an exercise-break from work, or duties at the office or in the home. Bounding provides the perfect answer. Some people moreover don't have the energy to jog or walk daily. You can take off your shoes and Rebound in your clothes (or underwear). Or, you can put on exercise shoes and/or exercise clothes to Rebound. There's no excuse for avoiding this activity.

Rebounding is so easy that even the most reluctant person will be enthusiastic about this very versatile form of exercise. In fact, a recent study by Dr. James White showed that almost twice as many people continue an exercise program of Rebounding than continue a jogging regimen after one year!

Exercising on the Bounder

The Bounder requires a "get-acquainted" session to familiarize yourself with it. The hand rails help keep your balance. If you have ever been on another Rebounder (or a trampoline), you will realize this scientifically-designed version is a new breed of exerciser. It's easy to develop a smooth rhythm and pace. You start out slowly rolling your feet in a heel-toe motion while keeping your feet on the mat. The high quality of this Bounder will aid your efforts and make the movement seem easy and natural. After a few minutes, you can rebound stiff-legged, allowing your body to just come off the surface. Soon, you will feel a pumping effect in your muscles. Tightening your upper body muscles (isometric contraction) will help exercise your entire body.

Rebounding, like all forms of exercise, requires a warming up period before you move on to your target heart rate exercises. My experience is that warmup periods are individual things. Two minutes may suffice for some people, ten minutes for others. Again, you must be in touch with your own body to know these distinctions. Now on to some rebounding exercises.

Rebounding for People Just Beginning an Exercise Program

If you have been inactive for some time, or if you exercise only once or twice per week, then you have to start slowly. Warm up by alternating walking and slow Rebounding. Try to achieve five minutes, then build up to fifteen minutes over a period of two to three weeks. Rebound at first every other day, then every day.

Once this is accomplished, you can exercise more vigorously. During this phase, exercising five times per week would be a good average. After warmup, increase your pace and lift your legs to imitate running. Alternate three minutes at a fast pace with three minutes at a slow pace. Rest three minutes between a couple of repeats. This will help both your cardiovascular (aerobic) conditioning and your muscle tone. During the exercise, let go of the handle bars and swing your arms in a horizontal plane to mimic the arm motion used in running. This action will help your coordination and improve upper body muscle tone.

A third phase for your rebounding program, which should occur after a few months, is to incorporate stiff-legged, low-height bounding. A slight bend in the knees is necessary to bound off the mat. This exercise will help your muscular development and your overall body strength.

Many of you will want to perform aerobic dance movement on the Bounder. Switch on the stereo and go at it! Improvise and determine what movements are most effective for you.

For the Overweight

This activity is an ideal exercise device for

people who are overweight. You can start out slowly and not suffer the pounding and joint stress caused by jogging or pedaling a stationary bicycle. Rebounding burns a lot of calories and works the muscles, too. The conversion of fat to muscle can take place quickly.

In the first phase of your exercise program, you should perform movements that keep both feet on the mat. The heel-toe shuffle (described above) will help you improve your aerobic capacity and get you ready for target heart rate activity.

When you can do at least ten minutes of alternate walking and jogging every other day, you can move on to Phase Two—alternating fast-pace and slow-pace movement with moderate leg lift for two ten minute periods, with five minute rest periods in between, at least five times per week. Phase Three exercises should include the muscle toning mentioned above and you should exercise at least five times per week. By then, you will have lost excess weight and be starting to improve your lean body mass (low body fat).

For Active People

You never get "rained out," making it an excellent exerciser for those days of inclement weather. It is also good for warming up and cooling down, before and after you run, jog, bicycle, and so on. And, since Rebounding works your entire body, you can use it to achieve peak conditioning.

Start out with a familiarization session, and then move on to an exercise regimen. You may want to do the alternating fast-pace, slow-pace, rest routine, or the muscle toning routine, both described earlier. Both these routines are very effective for building endurance and increasing circulation. It is also particularly effective on those days when soreness or stress from other exercise programs (such as weight training) is a barrier to working out.

For the Athlete

Rebounding can help improve athletic performance. These exercises affect several different forces your body is subjected to during exercise or competition; namely, acceleration, deceleration, and gravity. Your body has to adjust to these forces in order to control your movement. Every muscle in your body works and gets exercised. Moreover, your timing, coordination, and rhythm are all improved—skills that are both desirable and necessary in athletic performance.

Reaching peak condition requires not overdoing it, especially if you are working on an exercise regimen or aerobic and muscle-toning exercises. Supplement your regimen with one workout per day.

I feel that ten to twenty minutes every other day is adequate, if you use it during your entire training cycle. It can provide significant gains for the athlete who needs to relax and loosen-up, as well as for the endurance performer who needs to develop lean muscles.

Sports specific exercises can be adapted for the Rebounder. Ball sport athletes can perform twists and body stretches; and, aerobic sports athletes can reach a high level rhythm without stress to their bodies. You can experiment with various movements on the All American Rebounder to give you a higher level of performance in you respective sports.

For All

Rebounding is a perfect exercise for young and old. It does not stress the fragile bones and joints. It improves balance, coordination, and circulation. Rebounding is a healthful recreation activity for the entire family. Although I wouldn't prescribe rebounding as the only exercise program, I feel everyone should rebound as a *stress-relieving* recreational activity. Rebounding can help clear the mind, reduce tension, improve concentration, and promote enthusiasm.

157

For the Handicapped

Science says we all need exercise, and this is particularly true in the case of the handicapped. Physical therapy in the hands of a trained therapist or skilled family member is often a lifetime routine for the physically handicapped.

If you would like more information on Rebounding, contact the Rebound Fitness Society, whose address and telephone number are listed below. They will be happy to send you information concerning the availability of this product and how you may obtain it.

REBOUND FITNESS SOCIETY
P.O. Box 116
Department C
Canfield, Ohio 44406
(216) 533-5673

Why Rebounding is the Most Effective Exercise for your Better Health and Well-Being

Why Rebounding?

Exercise is essential for good health.

Fitness levels peak in your early 20's and normally decline as we age. But those who exercise regularly can be as fit at 85 as a sedentary person is at 20.

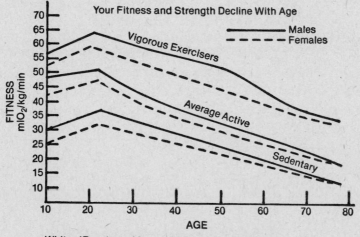

White, JR., adapted from UCSD faculty study, 1980.

159

The benefits of rebounding are legendary among the experts who have studied this popular new form of exercise.

Dr. James R. White in "Jump for Joy" states that when you rebound regularly for a sufficient length of time, every cell in your body changes and improves, providing increased endurance, aerobic capacity and cardiovascular enhancement. After NASA evaluated rebounding, they announced that rebounding exercise is 68% *MORE EFFI-CIENT* than jogging or any other activity.

Rebounding virtually eliminates injuries that are common to running, jogging, bicycling and rowing. The noted health authority William Fischer reports that exercise eliminates everyday stress and can help overcome depression. He states "exercise with the new rebounder improves secretion of important body hormones which help memory, learning and the sex drive."

160

Rebounding Provides Effective Exercise, and is Fun!

Using the rebounder burns up as much as 200 calories in ten minutes, and it is fun (see chart).

A year long study of various forms of exercise showed that 58% of participants rebounding were still bounding after one year—the highest percentage of any aerobic exercise tested! Moreover, exercising on the rebounder is the safest, injury-free exercise yet devised by man . . . And it is also extremely effective compared to any other form of physical activity.

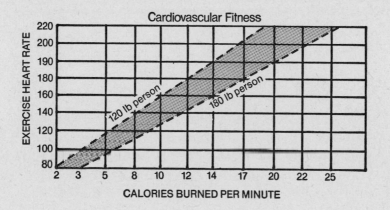

161

Chapter 7

Fit For Life Award Winning Recipes For Better Health

FISH FILET — A "DELIGHT FOR THE PALATE"

2 packages frozen fish filet	1 can mushrooms
	⅔ cup lowfat cheese
1 tbsp. butter	
a small can mandarins	

Remove the fish filet from the tinfoil, place on a heat-resistant platter with butter. Bake in the oven at 425° for 30-35 minutes. Drain the mandarins and mushrooms, and cube the Gouda cheese. Top the filet with the ingredients and brown 4-5 minutes, until the cheese begins to melt.

RED MULLET FILET IN ALUMINUM FOIL

2 lbs. red mullet filet	pinch of rosemary
juice from 1 lemon	3 peeled tomatoes
salt	½ cup baby Gouda cheese
1 large onion	½ bunch parsley
½ cup lean, smoked bacon	butter for greasing

Wash the fish, blot dry with a towel. Sprinkle with drops of lemon juice and lightly salt. Let soak through. Chop the onions, and cut the bacon into thin cubes, tomatoes into slices. Butter the tinfoil, arrange a layer of fish over it, cover with the bacon and onion cubes, and season with rosemary. Top with the tomato slices, and place the cheese slices over the tomatoes. Cover with the remaining fish filet. Cover the dish tightly with tinfoil, set in the oven, and bake at 375 °-400 ° for 20-25 minutes. Serve sprinkled with chopped parsley.

SPANISH CHICKEN CASSEROLE

4 chicken legs,	2 fresh green peppers
salt, pepper	4 peeled tomatoes
paprika, thyme	1 can petite peas (14 oz.)
3 tbsps. vegetable oil	1 cup cubed lowfat cheese
3 medium onions	
1 cup long-grain rice	
3 cups broth	

Thaw chicken legs in the refrigerator overnight. Rub the seasonings into the skin and cook in hot vegetable oil on all sides until golden brown. Cut the onion into rings and add to the pan. Saute until golden-yellow, and add the rice. Fill the pan with boiling broth. Let the rice simmer on low heat for 15 minutes. Wash the peppers and cut into strips, cut the peeled tomatoes into eighths and add to the rice. After 8 minutes, add the drained peas and cubed cheese. Combine carefully, season to taste and serve.

STUFFED CHICKEN

1 roasting chicken	½ tsp. caraway
pepper	2½ oz. cubed cheese
onion	2 tbsps. sherry
1¼ tbsps. butter	¾ cup water
3 oz. mushrooms	½ cup double cream
10 olives	salt to taste
3 large sweet gherkins	
1 tbsp. capers	
¼ cup raisins	
½ tsp. nutmeg	
½ teaspoon thyme	

Rub the chicken with pepper and saute the chopped onion in the butter. Stir in the washed, sliced mushrooms, sliced olives, sliced pickled gherkins, capers, raisins and seasonings. Simmer for 10 minutes and then stir in the cheese and the sherry. Stuff the chicken with this mixture and keep any leftovers for the sauce. Skewer the chicken to prevent the stuffing from coming out and grill on a spit for about one hour. Add the water to the remaining stuffing, heat through, stirring continuously. Finally, stir in the cream and season to taste.

CHICKEN IN AN EARTHEN POT

1 3-lb. chicken	3 onions
salt	1 bunch parsley
pepper	2 lbs. of canned corn
paprika	1 cup Gouda cheese
oregano	
9 oz. mixed dried fruit	

Remove the chicken from the package and let it thaw overnight in the refrigerator, covered. Then rub in the seasonings. Set an earthen pot in cold water for 20 minutes. Cut the onions into fourths, wash the parsley and stuff into the chicken. Close the opening with 2-3 pins. Drain the corn well, and cut the cheese into narrow strips. Layer the dried fruit, corn and cheese in the pot, and season with a dash of salt. Set the chicken on top, cover, and set into a cold oven. Set the oven to 400 degrees. Bake for 2 hours; uncover the last 10-15 minutes so that the meat will turn perfectly brown and crispy.

TOASTED CHEESE AND
CHICKEN SANDWICH

2 slices whole wheat bread	4 radishes
1 oz. grated Edam cheese	salt and pepper
1-2 oz. cooked chicken	

Sprinkle half of the grated cheese on one of the slices of toast, arrange the pieces of cooked chicken on top, cover with chopped radishes, sprinkle with a little salt and pepper and the rest of the grated cheese. Heat under broiler and then place the other slice of bread on top, if desired.

TOASTED CHEESE AND
MUSHROOM SANDWICH

1 oz. fresh mushrooms	salt and pepper
2 slices whole wheat bread	seasoned salt
2 slices Gouda cheese	2 green pepper rings

Saute the mushrooms in butter. Put a slice of cheese onto one of the slices of bread and arrange the mushrooms on top. Season with a little salt, pepper and seasoned salt, then cover with the rings of pepper and the second slice of cheese. Heat under broiler until cheese melts and then top with the second slice of bread.

TOASTED CHEESE
AND BANANA SANDWICH

2 slices whole wheat bread	1 tbsp. raisins or honey
2 slices Gouda cheese	pat of butter
½ banana	

Cover one piece of bread with a slice of cheese topped with sliced banana and garnish with raisins or honey, to taste. Complete the sandwich with the second slice of cheese and bread. Butter the outer side and grill in a frying pan as you would a grilled cheese sandwich.

SAUERKRAUT SALAD

1 large sour apple	4 oz. sour cream
lemon juice	salt
6 oz. sauerkraut	pepper
2 shallots	seasoned salt
2 rings of pineapple	tabasco sauce
1 tbsp. raisins	thyme

Chop the apple finely, sprinkle with lemon juice and add to the raw, finely shredded sauerkraut. Chop the shallots finely, cut the pineapple in small pieces, then mix the shallots, pineapple and soaked raisins into the sauerkraut. Beat the sour cream with a little salt and the seasonings. Toss through the salad ingredients.

WINTER SALAD

1 large carrot	salt
1 cucumber	pepper
1 apple	seasoned salt
juice of ½ lemon	ground paprika
2 pieces endive	tabasco sauce
8 oz. yogurt	

Wash and grate the carrot, and mix with the cubed cucumber, chopped apple, lemon juice and the finely sliced endive. Stir the salt and seasoning into the yogurt and mix into the vegetables.

171

BRABANTINE SALAD

	Dressing:
2 heads Belgian lettuce	
1 tbsp. raisins	1 cup yogurt
2 apples	2 tbsps. honey
1 small can mandarin wedges	½ tsp. sharp mustard
1 cup baby Gouda cheese	juice from 1 lemon
	juice from ½ orange
	few lettuce leaves

Wash the Belgian lettuce. With a sharp knife, cut a thin slice and carve out the bitter pulp. Separate the sprays and cut into strips lengthwise. Simmer the raisins somewhat. Cut the pared or unpared apples into small slices. Combine the Belgian lettuce, apples, mandarins, raisins and Gouda cheese cut into strips. Prepare the dressing with yogurt and other ingredients, and pour over the salad ingredients. Chill for 15 minutes before serving and serve in a bowl garnished with lettuce leaves.

CAULIFLOWER SALAD "EDAM"

1 medium cauliflower	Marinade:
juice from ½ lemon	4 tbsps. vegetable oil
1 small can baby peas	2-3 tbsps. vinegar
4 tomatoes	salt, pepper
1 cup Edam cheese	1 bunch parsley

Wash the cauliflower. With the head facing downward, lay in cold saltwater for 15 minutes. (Use 2 tbsps. salt for every 4 cups of water). Afterward set into boiling saltwater (1 tsp. salt for every 4 cups water) with the added lemon juice, and boil for 15 minutes. Remove the head with the skimmer, let it cook, and separate into rosettes. Thoroughly drain the peas on a sieve, and cut the tomatoes into eighths and the cheese into strips. Prepare the marinade dressing from vegetable oil, vinegar, seasonings and finely-chopped parsley, and pour it over the salad ingredients. Toss well but carefully and set aside for 15-30 minutes.

THICK BEAN SALAD

1 package thick beans	Dressing:
1 cup water	½ cup smoked lean bacon
pinch of salt	4 medium onions
¼ tsp. savory	2 tbsps. vegetable oil
14 oz. can peeled tomatoes	2 tbsps. vinegar
1 cup baby Gouda cheese	fresh ground pepper
	1 bunch parsley

Bring water to a boil. Add the unthawed beans with salt and savory and stew for 15 minutes, covered. Meanwhile cut the bacon into not-too-small cubes, and saute until glazed. Add the diced onions and saute until glazed. Add vegetable oil, vinegar and finely-chopped parsley to the bacon-onion mixture. Slice the cheese and add it to the mixture along with the warm beans and whole can of tomatoes with their juice. Combine carefully and let it set for ½ to 1 hour.

SAUERKRAUT SALAD "MANDARINO"

Dressing:	Salad:
1 cup yogurt	1 can mandarin oranges
1 tbsp. lemon juice	1 can sauerkraut
1 tbsp. mandarin juice	1 large apple
pinch of sugar	½ cup baby Gouda cheese
pinch of salt	

Prepare the dressing with yogurt and the mentioned ingredients. Lay the mandarins on a sieve and drain well. Chop the sauerkraut, if desired. Cut the apple into fourths, and then cut into thin slices. Cut the gouda also into thin slices, and toss the ingredients with the dressing. Season the salad to taste and serve immediately.

EPILOGUE

Without a healthy heart, little else matters. In fact, without good health, life doesn't seem worth living.

Good health is not something that just happens to people, as many of us once thought. Good health takes discipline, hard work and determination. But the rewards are like no other—life itself.

That's why more of us are taking direct control over our bodies. That's why more of us are learning all we can about how our bodies work and why certain habits are bad and others are good.

This book is intended to help you along the road to good health. It's one resource to use in your journey.

Throughout this book we explained how various products may make your quest for health easier. You should be able to find all of these products at your local health food store. If your favorite store doesn't carry a certain item, ask them to. Most retailers are more than happy to comply with special requests.

It is not wise to accept substitutes of a

similar nature, or a product that is "almost as good as" or "cheaper than."

Whatever the product, someone is bound to find a way to imitate it or produce it cheaper, very often at the expense of quality. Synthetic or chemically fertilized products are often substituted for natural or organic products. These manufacturers try to tell us they are just as good as the original, yet it's been proven there are great differences in quality between these products.

If for some reason you can't find the particular item to suit your individual needs or if you prefer shopping at home and avoiding the traffic and agitation, you can call or write the address listed below. *Biowell* carries the items mentioned in this book. Use the toll free number and the friendly and courteous telephone operators will help you in making selections.

By the way, if you are a retailer and would like to carry these products, call or write *Biowell*.

They also distribute to health food stores nationwide. They'll extend that same efficient courteous service to you.

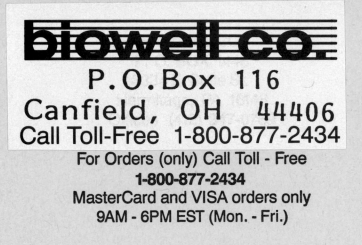

biowell co.

P. O. Box 116
Canfield, OH 44406
Call Toll-Free 1-800-877-2434

For Orders (only) Call Toll - Free
1-800-877-2434
MasterCard and VISA orders only
9AM - 6PM EST (Mon. - Fri.)

May good health be yours.

INDEX

ORDER FORM

Quantity Ordered	Book Title	Price	Total
	The Romance of Creative Healthy Cookery	18.95	
	How To Fight Cancer And Win	16.95	
	The Miracle Healing Power Through Nature's Pharmacy	19.95	
	How To Survive In The Hospital	12.95	
	Breakthrough in Arthritis	16.95	
	Mysterious Cause Of Illness And How To Overcome Every Disease From Constipation To Cancer	16.95	
	Eye Secrets To Better Sight	16.95	
	The Dr. Rinse Formula	9.00	
	Secrets To A Healthy Heart And Low Cholesterol	14.95	
	Miraculous Breakthroughs For Prostate and Impotency Problems	22.95	

Shipping & Handling Charges

$4.00 for one book
additional books, add $1.00

┌─ **For Extra Fast Service** ─┐
MasterCard and VISA orders only
☎ **Just dial (216) 533-1232**
8a.m.-5 p.m. (EST) Mon.-Fri.
Please have your card ready
No COD's please

Sub-Total	$
Shipping & Handling	$
Total	$
Ohio Residents add 5½% Sales Tax	$
Total Cost	$

I've enclosed a check or money order (sorry, no C.O.D.'s), in the amount of $_____
payable to **FISCHER PUBLISHING CORP.**

Please charge my account:
MINIMUM CHARGE ORDER IS $20.00   MasterCard ☐   VISA ☐

Please copy your card number   Exp. Date

Card Holder's
Signature_____

NAME _____ PHONE #(____)_____

ADDRESS_____

CITY _____ STATE_____ ZIP_____

FISCHER PUBLISHING CORP.
Box 368   Canfield, Ohio 44406
(216) 533-1232